"As a physician who is also a cancer survivor, I consider this book a true blessing! It's written in easy-to-read language and chock-full of information for navigating the rough waters of cancer. This book will make a huge difference for patients and their families."

Holly Johnson, M.D.
Florida Hospital Centra Care Clinic
Winter Springs, Florida

"Cancer—Now What? has transformed my wife's and my outlook and empowered us to move forward with greater focus and confidence. For patients and families seeking guidance, strength, and hope, this is the book you need!"

Jack
Family Member
Pebble Beach, California

"During a crisis like cancer, it's good to have a 'how-to' manual to guide you. That's why this book is so valuable—it's an excellent guidebook for patients and families dealing with cancer."

Jayson Neagle, M.D.
Assistant Professor
Feinberg School of Medicine, Northwestern University
Chicago, Illinois

"Cancer—Now What? is an amazing resource, filled with practical, useful information while offering compassion, encouragement, and hope. It's an incredibly helpful book for patients or their loved ones, including parents of a child or teen with cancer."

Heather Kaplinski, Ph.D.
Clinical Child/Adolescent Psychologist
Aspen, Colorado

"Any time you have questions, refer to this book. Look at the table of contents, find what you're wondering about, and turn to those pages. This book is packed full of valuable, reliable information that will guide you through the cancer journey."

Lyn Robertson, RN, MSN, DrPH
University of Pittsburgh Cancer Institute
Pittsburgh, Pennsylvania

"Cancer—Now What? is unique in how well it covers such a broad spectrum of clinical, spiritual, and psychosocial topics that can arise during the treatment of cancer. Patients, families, and caregivers will all benefit from this compassionate, well-written book."

Victor G. Vogel, M.D., MHS, FACP
Director, Breast Medical Oncology/Research
Geisinger Medical Center
Danville, Pennsylvania

"As I read it, I kept thinking, 'Yes, that's exactly how I feel!' and 'That's just what I needed to know!' It's spot-on in what it says and covers every key issue you'll likely face. This book is a priceless gift to all who read it."

Rita
Survivor
Boise, Idaho

"This book is so valuable. It's filled with understandable, need-to-know information that's grounded in the real-life experiences of patients, their families, and doctors and nurses. It's the most complete, caring, and reliable book on cancer I've ever seen."

Tom
Survivor
Boston, Massachusetts

"Cancer—Now What? covers a wide range of issues in a concise, understandable, helpful way. It's an excellent book for the person with cancer and also for family and friends wondering what they can do."

Ann Giddens
American Cancer Society, Retired
Abilene, Texas

"I've never encountered a book that offers as much helpful guidance after a cancer diagnosis. And with Dr. Haugk's warm, conversational tone, it's like a knowledgeable, caring friend has come over to help, right when you need it most."

David L. Charney, M.D.
Psychiatrist and Medical Director
Roundhouse Square Counseling Center
Alexandria, Virginia

CANCER
Now What?

CANCER
Now What?

TAKING ACTION, FINDING HOPE,
AND NAVIGATING THE JOURNEY AHEAD

KENNETH C. HAUGK, Ph.D.

Cancer—Now What?

Taking Action, Finding Hope, and Navigating the Journey Ahead

The purpose of this book is to provide those diagnosed with cancer and their loved ones with knowledge and practical ideas for dealing with cancer. To that end, every effort has been made to ensure that the information in this book is accurate and up to date at the time of publication. The information in this book is not, however, intended to replace the advice of a qualified, licensed medical professional. The author and publisher urge readers to consult with their own healthcare providers on any matters related to their health.

Neither the author nor the publisher makes any representations or warranties with respect to the information offered in this book; nor are they liable for any direct or indirect claim, loss, or damage resulting from use of the material in it. Those statements in this book that pertain to alternative or complementary treatments for cancer have not been evaluated by the FDA.

To those diagnosed with cancer,
the loved ones walking alongside them,
and the medical professionals
working on their behalf

CONTENTS

Acknowledgments vii

Introduction: You Are Not Alone ix

Part 1: What Do I Do Now?

1. A World Turned Upside Down 3

2. You're Not a Statistic 5

3. A Roller-Coaster Ride 7

4. One Enemy, Many Allies 9

5. Telling Others about the Cancer Diagnosis 11

Part 2: Dealing with the Emotional Dimension of Cancer

6. The Emotional Aftershocks of a Cancer Diagnosis 21

7. Accept and Express Your Feelings 25

8. Don't Feel Bad about Feeling Bad 29

9. Have a Good Cry 31

10. Feel Free to Get Angry 35

11. Feel Free *Not* to Get Angry 37

Part 3: Becoming Informed

12. The Value of Being Informed 41

13. Medical Questions to Ask and When to Ask Them 43

14. Where to Look for Information about Your Kind of Cancer 53

15. Network with People Who Have Been There 63

16. Keeping Track of Personal Medical Information 69

17. Thanking People Who Have Helped You Learn More 77

18. Updating People Who Have Helped You Learn More 81

Part 4: Understanding Medical Matters

19. Getting a Second Opinion 87

20. Clinical Trials 93

21. Pain Management 103

22. Side Effects 113

23. Palliative Care 121

Part 5: Alternative or Complementary Therapies

24. Defining and Describing Alternative and
    Complementary Therapies 127

25. Ask First 131

26. Three Categories for Considering Suggestions 133

Part 6: Working with and Relating to Your Medical Team

27. Bring Someone with You to Appointments 139

28. Take Notes 143

29. Focus Your Questions 147

30. Share Streamlined Information 151

31. The Gift of Empathy 153

32. Laughter Enhances the Best Medicine 155

33. Passivity Doesn't Work 159

34. Aggression Doesn't Work 165

35. Assertiveness Works 169

36. Be an Appreciator 175

37. Help Your Medical Team Help You 179

Part 7: Defining and Caring for Yourself

38. Don't Let Cancer Define You 185

39. Praise Yourself for Your Courage 191

40. Do Something Nice for Yourself 193

41. Go Easy on Yourself 197

42. Holidays and Other Celebrations 199

43. Have a Good Laugh 203

44. Forgive Others 207

45. Forgive Yourself 211

46. Accept Help 215

Part 8: Relating to Immediate Family

47. Cancer Upsets the Family Dynamic 221

48. Everyone Reacts Differently 227

49. Go Easy on Each Other 231

50. Share What You're Feeling 235

51. Ask Others How They're Doing 241

52. Listen Carefully 247

53. Create a Safe Place 251

Part 9: Relating to Friends and Extended Family

54. Keeping Family and Friends Up to Date 257

55. Some Relationships May Change 263

56. Seek Listeners, Not Lecturers 265

57. Find One or Two Triple-A Friends 267

58. Tell Others What You Need 271

59. Seeing Other People Go On with Their Lives 275

60. Say No 277

61. Say Yes 281

62. Ignore Raised Eyebrows 283

63. Avoid Toxic Individuals 285

Part 10: Additional Support

64. Find Kindred Spirits 291

65. Consider a Support Group 295

66. Share, Don't Compare 299

67. Be Open to Professional Counseling 301

Part 11: Spiritual Matters

68. The Spiritual Side of Dealing with Cancer 305

69. A Spiritual Roller Coaster 307

70. Be Totally Honest with God 309

71. Exercise Your Spirituality 313

72. Seek Out Spiritual Community 319

Part 12: Giving Back

73. Pay It Forward 325

74. Become an Advocate 329

Appendix

Chronological Diagnosis and Treatment Tracking Tools 333

Thank You 343

About the Author 344

About Stephen Ministries 345

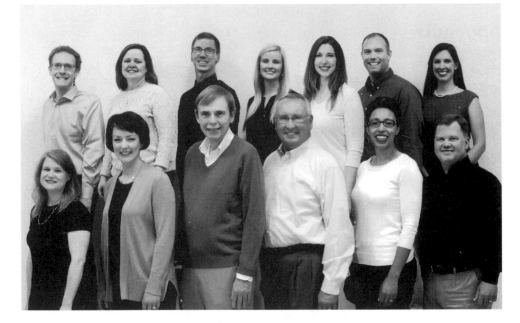

Members of the *Cancer—Now What?* Research Team

Front Row: Lori Kem, Kim Hoffer, Kenneth Haugk, David Paap, Janine Ushe, Kevin Scott

Back Row: Robert Musser, Pamela Montgomery, Joel Bretscher, Emily Noonan, Amity Haugk, Justin Schlueter, Rachel Remington

Not Pictured: Scott Perry, Jeanette Rudder, Gary Voss

ACKNOWLEDGMENTS

My name appears on the cover of this book, but that tells only part of the story. Many people played a significant role in bringing this book to you, and I'd like to thank them here.

The Research Team

I had the privilege of working with a talented and highly committed research team that contributed greatly to the quality of the book. The team members on the facing page put well over 35,000 hours into this project. Together, we:

- conducted 173 focus groups;
- interviewed 1,037 cancer survivors, loved ones of those diagnosed with cancer, and medical professionals;
- studied the comments and suggestions of thousands of readers; and
- engaged in many in-depth discussions about the best ways to make the book simple yet profound, exhaustive without being exhausting.

As we listened to the stories and wisdom of those who have personal or professional experience with cancer, our team grew even more dedicated to providing the most useful, encouraging, and effective resource possible.

Those on the Front Lines

I'm deeply grateful to the 2,741 survivors and loved ones whose firsthand knowledge and experiences enrich this book.

My gratitude also goes to the 820 medical professionals, in oncology and other fields, who shared their expertise and wisdom. They included oncologists and other physicians, surgeons, nurses, research scientists, pharmacists, and many others from a variety of disciplines.

All these individuals shared generously through in-person and phone interviews, written reflections and analyses, and group discussions. Their words, experiences, and insights brought additional substance, authenticity, and warmth to this book.

Those Who Provided Feedback on the Book

I'm indebted to the survivors, loved ones, and medical professionals who gave feedback on the book manuscript. These included:

- 2,125 people who read parts of the book as it was being developed; and
- 836 people who read the book from beginning to end after all the chapters were finished.

Their suggestions were invaluable and helped increase the overall usefulness of the book.

The Home Team

I appreciate the administrative skills of Emily Noonan, Sarah Hallstein, Ellen Garnett, and Tiffany Najbart, who organized and tracked thousands of documents, maintained personal contact with people giving feedback, and kept the entire project moving forward.

Many thanks to David Paap, Joel Bretscher, Kevin Scott, Robert Musser, Scott Perry, Jeanette Rudder, Stephen Glynn, and Gary Voss for editing the manuscript extensively. They helped me say exactly what I wanted to say, and they contributed significantly to the goal of putting together the most practical book possible for people with cancer and for their loved ones.

I'd also like to thank Kirk Geno for his excellent work designing the book cover and layout as well as typesetting the manuscript.

Finally, thanks to the proofing team of Robert Musser, Becky Bogar, Isaac Akers, Susan Jorgensen, and Maggie Schroeder for going over the final text with careful and attentive eyes.

On behalf of all those who contributed to this book, I am privileged and honored to send *Cancer—Now What?* out into the world. May it help you and your loved ones navigate the journey ahead.

You Are Not Alone

When my wife, Joan, was diagnosed with stage IIIC ovarian cancer, we were overwhelmed—and suddenly facing a lot we had to learn. Our emotions settled over time, and we did learn what we needed to know, but it was at times a slow and frustrating process.

When you're facing cancer, it's important to seize each opportunity and gain every advantage you can. The intent of this book is to help you be effective and efficient in dealing with cancer, whether it's you or a loved one who has been diagnosed. I want to equip you to navigate the challenges you may face and get the best possible care and treatment.

Joan and I learned much along the way. Working with her medical team, we were able to extend her life beyond expectations, help her live with purpose, meaning, and dignity—and give her the chance to hold our newborn grandson. My hope is to save you time and energy by sharing what we learned.

Collected Wisdom

What Joan and I learned is only part of this book. Together, a research team and I interviewed, surveyed, and conducted focus groups with 3,561 people who had experience with 81 different kinds of cancer. These individuals included:

- people who have had cancer;
- loved ones of those diagnosed with cancer; and
- medical professionals in oncology and other fields, some of whom have had cancer themselves or whose loved ones have had cancer.

This book incorporates their experiences and insights as well.

The Goal of This Book

This is a practical how-to book with the goal of helping those with cancer and their loved ones address the medical, emotional, relational, and spiritual challenges that cancer brings. Whether you read it cover to cover or move around from chapter to chapter depending on your needs at any given time, my desire is that this book will be a source of help and hope for you.

Standing with You

This book comes to you from people who have been there—people who, based on their personal or professional experience, are passionate about helping others facing cancer. That's certainly true for me, and it's true for all those whose wisdom, knowledge, and experience have been included in this book.

All of us stand with you. You are not alone.

—Kenneth C. Haugk

Part 1

What Do
I Do Now?

1

A World Turned Upside Down

"Those were very stressful days. First the shock and disbelief, then the fear. I felt like my whole world was crashing in on me."

The diagnosis of cancer changes everything. One minute you're leading a normal life. The next minute your whole world has been turned upside down.

Here's how some people described the time immediately after hearing a diagnosis of cancer:

- "I couldn't believe it. I just kept hoping someone would say it was a mistake."
- "I trembled all over and just couldn't stop crying."
- "I was in shock. My eyes glazed over, and my mind went blank."
- "Whatever the doctor said after that one word—*cancer*—might as well have been in another language."

Some people experience denial and disbelief. Others feel scared, sad, or angry. One man said, "I was furious that my own body, my own cells, had turned against me."

Here are two important things to know about this time.

First, whenever people receive news that shakes their world, they're likely to experience a whirlwind of emotions—and a cancer diagnosis for yourself or a loved one is often that kind of news. Many people say that the days after the diagnosis are among the worst in their lives. When all your plans for the future are suddenly thrown into question, it's only natural to feel that way.

Second, the initial turmoil and confusion eventually subside. Countless people who have had cancer or whose loved ones have had cancer will attest to this. A woman told me, "Right after my diagnosis, everything seemed so confusing, and I felt helpless. At first, I couldn't even hear or understand half of what the oncologist said. But over time my confusion faded, and I was able to think more clearly."

Let me offer these words of encouragement rooted in Joan's and my experience. Your mind will become clearer, and your focus will sharpen. You will become more knowledgeable about the kind of cancer you're dealing with and its treatments. You will learn much of the medical language that may seem so strange at first. You will gain a better understanding of the healthcare system and how to work with it.

It might not happen right away, but as you learn more, your uncertainty will decrease, your coping skills will kick in, and you will be ready to face this enemy called cancer.

2

You're Not
a Statistic

*"The statistics showed I had a 30 percent chance
of living five years. That was 27 years ago."*

In 1954, tiny Milan High School in southern Indiana competed for the state championship in boys' basketball. At the time, there was a single state title for all high schools in Indiana, with no divisions based on school size. Milan was facing schools over ten times its size. Statistically, it didn't seem to have a chance. But Milan defied the odds—and won the state championship.

That's just the way statistics are. They're helpful sets of numbers—data sorted into understandable patterns. They can indicate the likelihood of certain occurrences based on what's happened in the past. But they cannot predict your future.

At a conference, I met a clinical statistician who tracks, analyzes, and summarizes numerical data related to cancer clinical trials. He said, "Cancer statistics can be very helpful in summarizing data, shedding light on overall trends across groups, and planning treatments, but they can't forecast outcomes for specific individuals. Statistics are numbers—they aren't people."

Maybe you've seen or heard some statistics about cure rates or the percentage of people who beat your kind of cancer. Here are some points to keep in mind about such numbers:

- Statistics are based on a variety of factors, but they can't completely take into account your unique circumstances. As one man said, "I was diagnosed with a very rare cancer, and my doctor told me the long-term survival rate was very low. I responded, 'That may be so, but those other patients weren't me, and I'm gonna do whatever I can to beat this!'"

- Cancer statistics, even the most unsettling ones, include a number for those who live through the cancer. Whatever that number may be, you can decide to do everything in your power to be counted among those who live. A survivor shared, "Grim statistics became my motivator. They made me determined to fight even harder." A young man said, "My father was told that, with his type of cancer, he would probably live only six months or so. Well, he made up his mind to keep fighting and *really live* that six months, plus many months after that—adding up to 13 years so far!"

- Statistics are numbers. Don't give them any power over you by thinking they determine what will happen. An oncology nurse offered this encouragement: "Don't ever let percentages fool you into thinking you only have so long to live. Nobody can predict that. I frequently see patients who live well beyond what the numbers seem to suggest."

- Cancer statistics are based on what happened in the past. They don't dictate any individual's future. Research is ongoing, technology continues to advance, new treatments are becoming available, and many treatments are being refined and improved. This means your situation may be different from that of the people who had the same kind of cancer before you. A woman with cancer said, "My attitude has always been: Statistics are nothing more than numbers that summarize what has generally happened to others. Every case is different—mine is different, and so is yours. So don't be intimidated by numbers. Just live!"

Many cancer survivors have told me they set aside statistics and focused on their own unique fight against cancer. One said, "My oncologist mentioned statistics briefly, but I never worried too much about them. I was concerned with fighting and winning, not with what happened in the past." Another put it this way: "When *you* live, your survival rate is 100 percent. Any other percentage is irrelevant to you."

Remember the team from Milan High School. They didn't let the odds intimidate or define them. Instead, they gave their all to come out on top, regardless of the statistics. You can do the same—view statistics for what they are and focus on your own situation.

3

A Roller-Coaster Ride

"After my friend was diagnosed, she had lots
of ups and downs. During treatment, she felt
normal on some days and felt wiped out on others.
She had good test results and setbacks, until
eventually the cancer went into remission."

When Joan was sleeping after her initial surgery, I wandered into the hospital's cancer resource center and picked up an article titled "A Rough But Growing Experience" by Barbara Nichols, a cancer survivor. One section of the article caught my eye: "Prepared for a Roller-Coaster Ride." Here's what the author said:

> During chemo my brother-in-law told me that, with my diagnosis of cancer, I was also given a free ticket to the world's biggest and most frightening roller-coaster ride I'd ever take! And was he right. [My husband] Don and I found that with good medical news like "the CT scan is clear," we felt like soaring to the sky. But, with bad medical news, the roller coaster plummeted. To provide us some balance, we decided that whenever we had medical news we'd always say, "It's the bad news for today," or, "It was the good news for the day." By trying to put the news in the context of the day, on bad days we could hope that there would be other, better news on another day. On the good news days this approach gave us a proper perspective, so we were not overwhelmed when we got the bad news. The high "highs" and the low "lows" of the roller coaster were a little more evened out this way.[1]

1 Barbara J. Nichols, "A Rough But Growing Experience," *Coping with Cancer,* November/December 1997, p. 64.

This article told me what to expect with cancer: good news some days, bad news other days. Encouraging test results one time, disappointing results another. Such ups and downs happen to just about everyone with cancer.

One man told me what really helped him was to think of his treatment as an endurance event, not a sprint. He said, "I conserved energy by taking the good news with a grain of salt and shrugging the bad news off as a temporary setback, knowing I was in this for the long haul." Another survivor said, "One thing that helped me cope was knowing that I wasn't just going up and down—I was also moving *forward.* As difficult as things sometimes got, I focused my thoughts on the progress I was making, and that kept me from overreacting to the downs or the ups."

You can expect ups and downs based on the medical news you receive. Some news may be hopeful. Other news may leave you feeling discouraged. All the ups and downs of this roller-coaster ride, all the turns and zigzags that can jerk you one way and then another, are part of dealing with cancer.

It helps to know early on about the cancer roller coaster so you won't be caught off guard. Expecting the ups and downs, knowing that many people experience them, can help you handle them.

4

One Enemy,
Many Allies

*"At first, I wasted too much time and energy fussing
and complaining about people when they made things
difficult for me. But then I figured out that the best
thing I could do was to let go of that frustration and
stay focused on fighting the cancer."*

You have only one real enemy right now: cancer. Focus on defeating that enemy. As much as possible, try to treat every person you encounter as an ally.

Now, I'll admit that it isn't always easy to think of everyone as being on your side. Occasionally you may run into people who are just hard to deal with—people who treat you in ways that are inconsiderate or rude. When you're already carrying a heavy load, it's possible for their conduct to add to your burden.

But as tempting as it can be to spend a lot of time being upset with such people, it just isn't worth it. Doing so can be a real drain on your energy, and that energy is better spent dealing with the cancer. A woman I talked with described it this way: "This was a time when I needed to focus my strength on getting better, so I tried not to waste it on petty squabbles with other people."

A great way of relating is to treat people like the allies you need them to be, whether they're acting that way or not. Be as kind, gracious, and considerate as you can—even if someone's behavior can be unpleasant for you to deal with at times.

When you're facing cancer, it's good to have as many people on your side as possible. If you treat people as your allies, including those people whose actions are sometimes frustrating, they'll be more likely to give you the support you need. The more allies you have, the more effectively you can deal with your true enemy.

5

Telling Others about the Cancer Diagnosis

*"While waiting for the biopsy results,
I realized that one of the things I was
most afraid of was the prospect of having
to tell people that I had cancer."*

At first, perhaps only a few people will know about the cancer diagnosis. Eventually, though, you'll probably tell others—and it can be challenging to share such news. The purpose of this chapter is to help you with that challenge.

General Suggestions

Here are some thoughts about telling others.

Be realistic about how much you can do and when you can do it. You may not have the time or energy to tell everyone right away. Some people begin telling others immediately after receiving the diagnosis; others need time to let it sink in.

When you're ready to tell people, you might start with those you're closest to and then tell others as you feel up to it. One man with cancer said, "At first, I just told immediate family and a few close friends, making it clear that I didn't want them to tell anyone else yet. I needed some time before I was ready to let more people know." Others choose not to tell anyone beyond a small number of loved ones. Do what works best for you.

It's okay to let your emotions show. Strong emotions may surface as you speak to others. If so, you don't need to hold back. One person told me,

"Whenever I said the words, 'I have cancer,' I'd start to cry. It was a little embarrassing at first, but also therapeutic in a way. I found that people were very understanding and supportive."

Consider asking someone to be with you when you share the news. A number of people have told me they found it helpful to have a close friend or family member with them as they told others about their cancer. One woman said, "I really appreciated having my husband by my side when I let family or friends know about my diagnosis. He was clear-headed and able to answer questions when I was too upset."

Consider asking someone to tell others for you. The son of a survivor told me, "Mom asked me to give the news to the rest of the family, who lived across the country. She wanted to tell everyone herself, but she just didn't have the energy, so it was helpful for her not to have to repeat the conversation multiple times."

You don't need to share every detail with every person. Share only what you feel comfortable sharing and what you think is appropriate, given your relationship with that particular person. Some people may respond with questions about the diagnosis or what your next steps will be. If you feel comfortable answering questions, do so. Otherwise, say something like, "I'm not ready to talk about that just yet."

Set boundaries for what people may pass along to others. Tell people what information they may and may not share about the diagnosis. It's perfectly appropriate for you to define your expectations and communicate them to others.

Choose the best means of communication for the situation. You'll decide the best way to let each person know. One possibility is to tell others about the diagnosis in person, especially if you have a close relationship with them. Another is to tell people by phone. Choose what is most comfortable for you.

If you plan to tell others by phone and have a number of people to call, consider asking someone you trust to make some of the calls. This person could start the calls by saying something like, "Frank asked me to call because he wanted you to know right away. He would have called you personally, but he's dealing with a lot right now."

Decide whether or not you want to use email or social media to tell people about the diagnosis. I talked with a number of people who used email or social media to let friends and extended family members know about their cancer diagnosis. Some said it worked very well; others said it didn't, and they cautioned against communicating the diagnosis in this way. A number of them thought the news of their cancer diagnosis was too personal to be shared via email or social media. In a few instances, they described how their emails were mass-forwarded without their knowledge or how private information was copied and pasted onto blogs or social media for anyone to see.

As you consider communicating by email or social media, ask yourself whether the news might reach people you'd rather tell in person. Some survivors said they felt bad when loved ones they wanted to tell face to face found out about the diagnosis online.

If you decide to communicate online about the diagnosis, think carefully about what details to include, because you can't be sure who will end up seeing them. Also, specifically state whether or not you want any of your information shared. Then realize that in spite of your precautions and requests, what you say electronically may end up being shared more widely than you intended.

Consider the time and place. One couple told me, "We told our son at a restaurant over lunch, but that turned out not to be a good choice. He got very emotional, and he was embarrassed that it was in public. Then he went back to work and had a lot of trouble holding it together for the rest of the day. In hindsight, we should have told him in private when he would have had time to process the news."

Recognize that people might respond to the news in many different ways. One person gave this advice: "Don't be surprised by the ways others react when you tell them about your cancer diagnosis. You may have had all kinds of difficult feelings when you first heard the diagnosis, and they might experience similar feelings."

People may respond with tears, confusion, optimism, fear, a torrent of questions, shocked silence, or something else entirely. Some people might rally to your side immediately. Others might need time to fully grasp the news before they respond.

A few people may become distraught upon hearing the news, and that can be hard for you to deal with. As one survivor said, "Some people really freak out, and you might end up thinking that you have to take care of them instead of the other way around." The news about the cancer can be very distressing, but don't pressure yourself into being a caregiver for others at this time in your life. If it's someone you want to comfort—such as a child or another close family member—and if you feel up to it, by all means do so. But as you are dealing with cancer, it's important to focus on caring for yourself. Someone who is especially upset by the news may need to find another friend or confidant to listen and care for him or her. You don't have to take on that responsibility.

Go easy on yourself. You don't need to worry about every detail of telling other people. If some people are unhappy with the way you told them, how long it took you, or whom you told before telling them, don't blame yourself.

Meet your own needs. Above all, as you tell others about the cancer diagnosis, do what's best for yourself based on:

- how much energy you have;
- how close you are to the person you're telling; and
- what you're most comfortable with.

Suggestions for Telling Specific Groups

In addition to those general guidelines, here are ideas for sharing the news with particular groups of people.

Adult Family Members

Many people start by telling the adult family members they're closest to. Family members are often deeply affected by the diagnosis, so it can be good to let close family know right away. They can become an indispensable source of help and support.

Some people told me that they saved emotional energy by gathering several family members and breaking the news to them all at once instead of one at a time. Others found it easier to tell family members one by one so they could respond to each person's emotions and questions individually.

Friends

When you tell friends about the diagnosis, it gives them the opportunity to show their friendship by caring for you. The husband of a woman with cancer said, "When I told my best friend, his first reaction was shock, but almost immediately his second reaction was, 'What can I do to help?' He and his wife were a constant source of encouragement and were there to give practical help when we needed it. Knowing that they cared was a real lift for both of us."

You don't have to tell all your friends immediately. At first, you might want to tell only one or two individuals you are particularly close to—the friends whose help and support you need the most. Over time, as you feel more comfortable sharing, you might tell others.

Teenagers

When you're ready to share the news with teenagers, consider the following suggestions. These points generally apply to telling adults as well, but they're especially important to keep in mind with teenagers.

Share Openly and Honestly

Give as many details as you feel comfortable sharing, also considering what the teenagers seem comfortable hearing. Invite them to ask questions anytime they come to mind.

Invite Them to Respond

After you've shared the news and answered any questions, encourage teenagers to tell you about their feelings and worries. They may feel anxious and unsure about what's going to happen next. They might wonder how all this will affect their lives as well as yours.

Some teenagers may find it difficult to share feelings, while others might express a range of intense emotions. If you express your feelings openly, it can help them feel more comfortable sharing. Check in with them after they've had time to process what they're thinking and feeling.

Respect Their Privacy

Even as you encourage teenagers to open up to you, also respect their privacy. Suggest that if they're uncomfortable talking with you about anything, they might talk with others such as trusted relatives, friends, teachers, counselors, members of a spiritual community, or peers in a support group. A woman told me, "My daughter was in high school at the time, and she had trouble opening up to me about my cancer. Thankfully, her church youth group and high school counselor gave her the outlets she needed for her feelings."

Provide Clear Boundaries for What to Share

Establish boundaries for what teenagers may share, especially on social media. Many teenagers regularly use social media to communicate with friends and to generate support when they're going through tough times. But if you'd rather not have your information shared so widely, let them know. One man said, "I decided to call each of my grandchildren to personally tell them about my diagnosis. But one of the first grandchildren I called posted about it online right away, and then a couple of the others saw the post before I could call them. In retrospect, I should have told them I'd prefer they not share the news that way."

Give Them Ways to Help

Teenagers might ask you what they can do to help. If so, suggest responsibilities they would be able to handle—perhaps tasks that you would normally take care of yourself. Being able to support you in specific, tangible ways often gives teenagers some sense of control over the situation.

Children

Bringing up the diagnosis with younger children can involve unique challenges. Here are some thoughts about how to tell them.

Do Tell Them the News

Children may feel distressed or confused when they hear about a cancer diagnosis, and it may be hard to tell them. But not telling them the news can often cause children even more anxiety. They will probably sense that something's wrong, even if you don't say anything about it. Then, because they don't know the details, their imagination can take over, and what they imagine may be far worse than reality. Also, children might overhear the news or learn it from someone else, which can intensify their fears and damage their trust. When you tell them the truth as soon as it's appropriate, you can strengthen their trust and help them cope with their fears.

Provide Information Appropriate for the Child

Share a level of information that's appropriate to each child's age and maturity. The older the child is, the more details you may want to share. But be sure to follow the child's lead, and don't try to answer questions he or she isn't asking.

With younger children, you'll probably need to share more generally: "I have a sickness called cancer. My doctor is going to give me medicine, but I'm probably going to be feeling sick for a while." One survivor said, "Young children don't need all the details. They just need to know that they're safe and loved and that everyone is doing their best to help their loved one get better."

Often children are concerned about how the diagnosis is going to affect them. It can help to share ways that things might change, such as:

- "Sometimes your aunt instead of your mom will pick you up from school."
- "I wish I could coach your soccer team this year, but I won't be able to. I'll try to come to as many games as I can, though."
- "Grandpa says he's sorry, but he won't be feeling well enough to take you to the amusement park this summer. But we'll still be going to visit him, and we'll find something fun we can do with him."

If there might be side effects the child would notice, such as hair loss during chemotherapy, let the child know about them in advance.

Sometimes younger children may be able to take in only part of what you've planned to say. If you sense that this is the case, it might be best to save the rest for another conversation.

Listen

After you've told a child what's going on, take time to listen, not only to what the child says but also to the meaning behind the words. Welcome any questions and answer them honestly and patiently, even if he or she asks the same questions over and over.

You may want to ask the child what he or she knows about cancer. Depending on the child's age, you might ask, "Have you heard of cancer before? Do you know what cancer is?" Pay attention to any possible misunderstandings or worries you can clear up, such as thinking that the cancer is somehow his or her fault or that it's contagious. Then share the truth to help address those fears.

Give children every chance to say what they're thinking or feeling, and let them know that their feelings are okay. Invite them to talk whenever they want or need to.

Let Other Adults in the Child's Life Know

Keep in mind that the diagnosis can affect a child's emotions and behaviors in everyday life. It's a good idea to inform other adults who relate to the child—such as childcare providers, teachers, coaches, school counselors, Scout leaders, religious leaders, and others—so they can be aware of what's going on, offer support, and let you know about any changes in the child's behavior.

A child psychologist who works with families affected by cancer told me, "Sometimes I'll help families write a brief note for teachers or coaches. It will say, 'This is the message we've shared with our child,' and then summarize what the child has been told. Teachers and coaches sometimes wonder, 'I know about the diagnosis, but how much does the child know, and what should I say or not say?' Telling them what the child knows can help."

How Children May Respond to the News

Children might not display a strong reaction to the news at first. In particular, young children sometimes deal with stressful news without a lot of emotion. One young mother recounted, "My son was six and my daughter was four. We sat them down, and I explained that I had cancer and that I might lose my hair because of the chemotherapy. My son said, 'You'll look just like Uncle Bill,' who is bald. My daughter asked, 'Can you paint my fingernails?'"

Children may want to help as the family deals with cancer. Let them assist in ways they can manage. Children often like to do what they can, and you can help them by letting them help you.

Children's responses to cancer depend in large part on what they observe in their parents and other adults. You'll help them by being confident while honestly expressing your emotions. You don't need to be stoic or conceal your feelings around children; if you need to shed tears, do so. By being realistic and emotionally honest, you let children know it's okay for them to be open about how they feel.

Above all, give children lots of love—for their sake and for yours.

Additional Resources That Can Help with Telling Children

The American Cancer Society (cancer.org) and the National Cancer Institute (cancer.gov) provide online and printed resources that answer a number of questions about telling children about a cancer diagnosis.

Telling Others Builds Support

Telling people about the cancer diagnosis is a key step in building strong support. People can't pitch in if they don't know what's going on. As one survivor pointed out, "Your friends and family want to be your support system—they want to be a part of this with you. Telling them about the diagnosis lets them in and invites them to help."

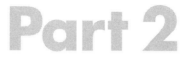

Part 2

Dealing with the Emotional Dimension of Cancer

6

The Emotional Aftershocks of a Cancer Diagnosis

"After my diagnosis I experienced denial, fear, panic—like a dark cloud covering everything— and the feeling that the world was out of sync. Then anger and frustration, followed by bitterness, resentment, and isolation."

Just as aftershocks can follow a big earthquake, you and your loved ones may feel emotional aftershocks following a cancer diagnosis. Many different feelings can come one after another or several at once.

Kinds of Emotional Aftershocks

This chapter describes some emotions people might experience when facing cancer. Subsequent chapters in this section will offer ideas for handling those feelings.

Keep in mind that each person is unique and will react to a cancer diagnosis differently. You may not experience all the emotions listed here, and you may feel others that aren't listed. Also, there's no set timetable for feelings; different emotions can come right after diagnosis or later on. Eventually, though, you'll probably encounter at least some of these feelings.

Shock and Disbelief

A cancer diagnosis can leave people feeling numb, in shock and disbelief. It can feel unreal, especially at first. A person's initial response may be, *This just can't be true!*

Right after the diagnosis, people often feel paralyzed and unable to act. As one survivor put it, "You hear the diagnosis, and all at once it's the roar of a tidal wave. No other sounds get in. The doctor is still talking, but you aren't hearing a thing."

A family member of a person with cancer reported a similar experience: "After my sister told me she had cancer, she continued on for a couple of minutes, until I finally said, 'Hold on a second. I haven't heard a thing you said since the word *cancer.*'"

Fear

It's natural to feel fear at any time after the diagnosis—anything from vague anxiety to all-out panic.

Some people have heard disturbing stories about the impact of cancer and its treatments. Others have watched family or friends struggle with cancer. Many have also seen the effects of cancer dramatized in TV shows and movies or described on the internet. Such experiences can add to a person's fear.

A cancer survivor told me, "Fear was a major struggle for me. A friend of mine had cancer about 10 years before I was diagnosed, and I was terrified at the thought of going through what she experienced."

Anger

Cancer is a huge intrusion in people's lives, and anger is a natural reaction. People may feel angry at the cancer, themselves, their body, family members, their medical team, God, or just about anyone or anything else. One person said, "I couldn't stand how unfair it all was. I had done everything I could to stay healthy, and my body betrayed me anyway."

Guilt

Sometimes cancer leaves people feeling guilty. They may wonder whether they did something to cause the cancer, or they may feel responsible for creating upheaval for their family and friends.

A woman shared this about her feelings of guilt: "The things some people said really made me feel like it was all my fault, as if I had caused my own cancer. Others seemed to be implying that if I didn't have a full recovery, it was because I wasn't positive enough. That made the guilt even worse."

Loneliness

People with cancer sometimes experience a sense of loneliness and isolation. They may believe that no one else really understands what they're going through. Friends or family members may try to be unwaveringly positive and upbeat, but that can actually prevent those with cancer from sharing how they really feel. It may leave them with the impression that they have to keep their suffering to themselves.

People with cancer and their loved ones may at times try to shield each other from difficult feelings by not talking about the situation. This lack of communication can result in even more feelings of loneliness.

Some friends or family members may pull away from the person with cancer because they don't know what to say or how to act. One survivor commented, "My family was in shock. They were afraid. They didn't know how to respond to me. I felt so alone." At times, people find that the less they talk about their cancer, the more they think about it—and the more isolated they feel.

Loss and Grief

Cancer can trigger a number of significant losses, such as the loss of health, physical functioning, independence, ability to work, a sense of normalcy, or future plans. These losses can bring grief and affect people in many different ways, including sadness, crying, and a feeling of listlessness. One person shared, "For a while after the diagnosis, I felt like all of my dreams were gone. I was an emotional wreck."

Sometimes the loss hits especially hard and leaves a person in a fog, making it difficult to engage with others. One man told me, "When I first learned about my diagnosis, I experienced mourning. It felt as though everything I enjoyed had been taken away from me."

Depression

Cancer can lead to depression. Sometimes people become so deeply depressed that they are unable to address their own basic needs. They may not be able to get out of bed, get dressed, or eat well. They may even become suicidal. If you see signs of depression like these, talk with your medical team.

Helplessness

After a cancer diagnosis, people can feel helpless—as if they've lost control over much of life. A business executive shared, "Professionally, I manage large numbers of people in massive projects. I'm used to being in control. All of a sudden, I had very little control of my own body and had to depend on others."

The Stress of a Cancer Diagnosis Can Magnify Feelings

During stressful times, feelings can be magnified, and people may react more strongly than usual to situations that otherwise wouldn't affect them much. This can be especially true following a cancer diagnosis, both for the patient and for loved ones.

A clinical psychologist said, "Everything having to do with cancer—including the diagnosis, the day-to-day challenges, and the medications and other treatments—can affect your emotional state. Your feelings and responses may be different from what you're used to."

Anyone May Experience Emotional Aftershocks

The emotional aftershocks of a cancer diagnosis can be challenging. It often helps to know that many people experience such feelings and are unsettled, at least for a while. The following chapters can help you deal with these emotional aftershocks as they occur.

7

Accept
and Express
Your Feelings

*"It was such a relief when I could
drop the mask and just say to someone,
'Right now, this is what I'm feeling.'"*

The previous chapter described how people with cancer—and those who stand alongside them—often experience a wide range of feelings. People may wonder, *How do I deal with all these emotions?*

A good starting point is to know that feelings are neither right nor wrong—they just are. People can't choose the feelings they have or when they will occur. But they can choose what to do with them. They can try to hide or deny feelings, or they can accept and express them.

Hiding Feelings

Sometimes people pretend that difficult feelings aren't there. They attempt to push the feelings down, hold them in, or ignore them. They hope that if they don't think about what they're feeling, maybe the emotions will just go away.

People might hide or deny their feelings for many different reasons:

- "I was taught to keep a stiff upper lip no matter what."
- "I didn't want people to feel sorry for me, so I didn't share much."
- "Everyone expects me to be strong, so I can't show raw emotions."
- "I was afraid that if I let my feelings out, I'd lose control."

- "I had so many responsibilities competing for my attention that I kept putting off dealing with my feelings."
- "I grew up in a family where the only feelings allowed were tough ones like anger."

Problems with Hiding Feelings

Dealing with feelings may be difficult, but trying to avoid them isn't the answer. The more that people hold in their feelings, the more those feelings can end up controlling them. No matter how or why people attempt to hide them, those feelings don't go away. Their power can build up until it wears people down or causes them to erupt—to speak or behave in ways they later regret.

The wife of a man with cancer told me, "My husband held his feelings inside until they exploded in a sudden burst of anger and he kicked a hole in the drywall in the back of the garage. I wanted to get it fixed, but he said, 'Let's leave it for a while. It'll remind me of what happens when I try to just tough it out instead of talking about what's going on.'"

Keeping feelings inside takes a lot of energy—more than it would take to express them. One person shared the following reflection:

> "When I tried to keep my difficult emotions inside, I couldn't stop thinking about them. The effort stressed me out and wore me down, which was the last thing I needed when I was already ill. Then an oncology social worker told me that it's important to get all those feelings out—the anger, fear, guilt, and sadness. Otherwise, they can consume you. That was great advice."

Accepting and Expressing Feelings

Rather than hiding or denying the feelings that cancer stirs up, it's far more helpful to accept and express them.

One time during Joan's fight with cancer, a friend asked me how I was doing. I told him, "Crappy." He responded, "Then *be* crappy." Those were encouraging words for me. I was feeling crappy, and it was all right to feel that way. I didn't have to fake it for anyone.

Accepting and expressing feelings won't necessarily happen in that order. Sometimes you accept a feeling first and then feel comfortable letting it out. Other times you might start by expressing the feeling and only afterward discover that you're able to accept it.

A survivor told me, "For a while, I had a hard time admitting my fears about cancer. But then, when I was talking to a friend, I found myself pouring out everything I was scared of. I stopped and thought for a moment, and then I said, 'I guess I'm really scared.'"

Benefits of Accepting and Expressing Feelings

Accepting and expressing your feelings can be especially beneficial when you're dealing with cancer.

- It can remove the pressure that comes from trying to mask feelings, clearing the way for sharper thinking and better decision making.

- When others know what you're going through, they can support you most effectively.

- Opening up to others about feelings can strengthen relationships.

Holding feelings inside tends to make life more difficult for everyone involved. Recognizing those feelings and letting them out, on the other hand, can make life easier for you and those around you.

Ways to Express Feelings

People express their feelings in different ways. Cancer survivors and their loved ones have found the following helpful.

Talking. One of the most common and effective ways to express feelings is to talk about them—to tell another person what's going on inside. People may talk about their feelings with:

- loved ones
- trusted friends
- a support group
- a mental health professional
- a pastor, chaplain, or other spiritual leader
- God

Each of those kinds of sharing will be covered more fully in later chapters. One woman said:

> "I was really scared, and at first I stuffed my feelings down way too much. But slowly I started letting them out, a little at a time. I mostly shared with another mom at the kids' play group; she always paid attention and didn't take over the conversation. She was just what I needed to get my emotions out: a friend who would listen, listen, listen!"

A nurse told me:

> "On the surface, I was very matter-of-fact about things and focused almost entirely on medical issues with Dad's cancer. On the inside, though, my heart was breaking. A fellow nurse and I had a long talk, and I was able to tell her about the tension I was struggling with. It was such a relief to talk to someone who understood how hard it can be for a nurse to deal with a loved one's serious illness."

Crying. People may get their feelings out through their tears. A woman with cancer said, "After coming home from a round of tests, my husband, daughter, and I just embraced in the garage without a word and cried together. Then we took a deep breath and were able to discuss the test results with more clarity. It was such a freeing moment."

Writing. Some people process their feelings by writing about them in a journal. Others express their emotions by writing letters, perhaps to a trusted friend or even to God. Whatever form the writing takes, it can be a safe and effective way to connect with and release emotions. A man who had cancer said, "My mind was fixed on all my fears and worries, which replayed in my head over and over. I was finally able to let go of them when I wrote them all down in a journal and then put it away until I needed it again."

Writing, then talking. Writing about feelings can open the door to talking about them. One person said, "Putting my feelings on paper helped me be honest with myself, which made it easier to be honest with others."

Creative outlets. Some people express their feelings through activities like drawing, writing a poem, or making crafts.

Physical activities. At times people might be able to release feelings through physical activity. The husband of a survivor said, "My wife swims regularly. She says that exerting herself in the pool helps her pour out her anger, stress, and anxiety." Although not everyone with cancer can engage in more vigorous physical activities, lighter activities such as taking a walk, stretching, or doing yard work can be ways to get difficult feelings out.

These are just some ideas. There's no one-size-fits-all approach to expressing feelings; it's about what works best for you.

Accepting and expressing feelings can benefit you and your loved ones. It can keep you focused, energize you, and pave the way for healthy relationships.

8

Don't Feel Bad
about Feeling Bad

*"Sometimes I was angry, scared, sad, and confused.
I knew that this was fairly normal for someone with
cancer, so I just felt what I felt."*

Dealing with cancer will most likely involve emotional highs and lows. There may be times when you're feeling pretty good. But there will probably be other times when you're feeling pretty bad. What do you do then?

Just allow yourself to feel what you feel. Don't feel bad about feeling bad.

In the book *Don't Sing Songs to a Heavy Heart,* I talk about "pink thinking"—the common, but mistaken, expectation that suffering people need to think positively and reject any negative feelings:

> Pink thinking is optimism run amok. Pink thinking denies the reality of an individual's suffering and glosses over the hurting person's pain.[1]

Putting pressure on yourself to feel better—thinking, *I shouldn't be sad or upset right now, I need to be positive*—will probably make you feel worse. One person told me, "Forcing myself to be positive, when that was the farthest thing from my mind, wore me out physically and emotionally."

Of course, some days will be better than others. Maybe you've just recovered from one treatment, the next is still a while off, and today feels like a really good day. By all means, enjoy that day. But if you're not having a good day, don't pressure yourself into faking happiness or pretending everything's fine.

An important reason to allow yourself to feel bad is that when you do, you may actually start to feel a bit better. Many people naturally feel sad and

---

1 Kenneth C. Haugk, *Don't Sing Songs to a Heavy Heart: How to Relate to Those Who Are Suffering* (St. Louis: Stephen Ministries, 2004), p. 115.

grieve the losses that come with a cancer diagnosis, and suppressing those feelings uses up a lot of energy. Allowing yourself to accept and express difficult feelings can help you relax a little and let go of them.

One survivor told me, "I don't always have to be upbeat. When I feel sad, I let myself cry. That helps me put one foot in front of the other and continue my journey. Then, when days are good, I'm free to enjoy them."

Another shared how she made it through the days when she felt really bad: "I would call up my best friend and tell her I was having a blue day. She would say, 'Start a pot of coffee brewing—I'm on my way.' Talking with her always helped."

However, if you just keep feeling worse and worse, or if your feelings begin to get in the way of daily life or your cancer treatments, talk with your medical team.

Dealing with cancer, whether your own or a loved one's, is tough enough. Dealing with cancer *and* trying to fake your feelings is even tougher. Give yourself a break and feel your feelings—whatever they may be.

9

Have a
Good Cry

*"After I was diagnosed, my wife and I held in our
tears, each trying to protect the other from the pain.
I remember the day we finally cried together.
The tears just flowed, and it felt good."*

Cancer can hit hard and hurt terribly. Many people have told me about one way they've dealt with the emotional pain of cancer: by letting their tears flow.

Crying can bring emotional healing. Painful feelings that stay buried and unexpressed can build up over time and cause additional problems. Shedding tears is a good way to release those feelings. A cancer support group leader said, "Befriend your tears. During the trial of cancer, they're a pathway to emotional health. Each tear releases pent-up feelings of hurt, fear, self-pity, and frustration that could otherwise fester inside."

For Some People, Tears Flow Easily

Some people find that crying comes naturally. One survivor told me, "Throughout my treatment, I cried whenever I needed to, sometimes because of the physical or emotional pain or fatigue, other times because I felt for the people around me. My husband was able to cry too. Tears really are healing!"

For Others, Tears Don't Come as Naturally

Other people don't cry as easily. One person said, "I don't cry often. I just have a hard time opening the floodgates."

People may feel uncomfortable crying. Perhaps they were taught that tears are undignified or a sign of weakness or self-pity. Or they may find it hard to cry because of who they are or how they're wired. Even when they feel sad, their tears don't come easily. Some people find that other ways of handling emotions work better for them.

But cancer may bring tears to people who don't often shed them. A man confided that he had always avoided crying—but then, after an exhausting round of treatment, he found himself weeping. He said, "Cancer still stinks, and the treatment is still tough, but crying actually did help me feel better."

Find a Safe Place to Cry

If you think crying might help, but you find it difficult to do, look for a safe, private place to cry, such as the bedroom, the shower, or a parked car. One person said, "When I needed to cry, I would go for a walk. It would get me out of the house, and I could be alone and have a good cry. By the time I got back, I was feeling relieved and relaxed." Another told me, "After we left the surgeon's office, my wife and I were overwhelmed with emotion. So we found a secluded spot, held each other, and wept." Still another explained that her safe place was at home with her golden retriever: "I'd let him up onto the sofa, put my arms around his neck, stroke his fur, and just cry. It always made me feel better."

Find Safe People to Cry With

Sometimes finding a safe place is about being with the right people—those you feel safe sharing your emotions with. Your tears may flow more freely when you're with a loved one or a trusted friend. A woman told me this story: "I had cancer when I was 13, and one evening I was throwing up over and over from chemotherapy. Dad was holding the bowl, and when I looked up, I saw that he was crying. He said, 'I would trade places with you if I could.' That's when I started crying too."

On the other hand, feeling unsafe with someone can put the brakes on tears. A man with cancer said, "When I'm with certain people, you're not going to see me cry—the trust level just isn't there. But with the right people, I can let it out."

Just Cry

Of course, you may need to cry right where you are—at just about any time or any place, without warning. Go right ahead. Don't let other people deter you. When cancer invades, you have every right to let your emotions out.

One man said, "My coworker had cancer and was struggling to appear strong for his wife and girls. One day, it was only the two of us in his office, and he just dissolved into tears. He needed to let it all out right then and there."

If your crying becomes debilitating and begins to interfere with your ability to eat, sleep, work, or do other daily tasks, talk with your medical team. Otherwise, letting your tears flow can be a helpful thing to do.

All this isn't to say that you *have* to cry. But if you feel like crying, don't hold back your tears.

10

Feel Free
to Get Angry

*"Sometimes I just needed to vent—to rant and rave,
to say out loud how mad I was and how unfair things
were. Getting my anger out gave me strength."*

Cancer can make you angry. But many people are uncomfortable with anger. They may have been taught that anger is bad and that expressing it isn't something nice people do. They might think, *If I were a better person, I'd be able to deal with cancer without feeling so furious about it.* They may believe expressing their anger about cancer would show a loss of self-control. They may worry about what others would think. Or they might have heard about people who seemed to handle cancer with unflappable calm—and they believe they should do the same. For reasons like these, people may deny their anger or try to keep it hidden.

But bottling up or ignoring these feelings can cause more harm than good. If anger continues to build up, it can unexpectedly erupt like a volcano, possibly hurting others and leaving you feeling guilty or embarrassed.

So go ahead and let yourself feel angry at times. After all, there's a lot about cancer that can make a person feel that way, and expressing it is much better than suppressing it. But try to do so in constructive ways.

Ways to Deal with Anger

Dealing with anger constructively can relieve stress and lighten your burden. Here are some ways to do this.

Talk about Your Anger

One of the best ways to deal with anger is to find a person to talk to—someone you trust to listen and accept whatever you have to say (see chapter 57, "Find

One or Two Triple-A Friends"). Letting it all out with this kind of person can be an immense relief. As one person with cancer said, "Not everyone can handle your anger or your raw emotions. But the right person will feel honored that you trust him or her with your feelings."

A nurse who had cancer told me:

> "I remember being at church for an evening service when I was filled with the worst anger I've ever had. My pastor noticed I wasn't myself, and we talked after the service. I was able to let it all out, including some words I don't normally use. It turned out that it helped a lot to talk about how mad I was."

Find a Safe Place to Express Your Anger

On occasion, you may choose to hold off expressing your anger until you're in a place where you feel safe venting it. One woman whose husband had cancer said, "We got bad news from some test results, and we were shocked and upset. We waited until we were alone in the car, and then we let out all our anger yelling at the cancer before driving home. It was good for both of us to air out those feelings, but we needed privacy."

Focus Your Anger

Anger can be an energizer and motivator. When you're really angry, it can get you thinking, *I'm going to get this cancer out of my body!* Directing your anger toward the cancer can give you the focus and drive to fight back.

A cancer survivor told me, "It's absolutely okay to be angry at cancer. It's completely unfair, with the cancer lying and cheating to get the upper hand, all while you're fighting as hard as you can. Being angry is a logical response. I used that anger to direct everything I had toward beating the cancer."

If You Need Help

If you're having an especially difficult time dealing with your anger, or if your anger is hurting you or others, talk with your medical team.

Anger isn't something to hide, bury, or be ashamed of. Anger is normal, and letting it out appropriately is okay—even good for you. This is true throughout your life, but especially when you're dealing with cancer.

There are also times, however, when you might choose *not* to get angry. The next chapter talks about when and how that might happen.

11

Feel Free *Not* to Get Angry

"During my treatment, I've learned not to get upset over the little things. The best thing I can do for myself is to focus my energy and attention on job number one: fighting cancer."

It's natural to get angry about cancer, and it's helpful to get your anger out. I've heard people let loose with some strong, colorful words about cancer, and I agree with them 100 percent. Feel free to let that anger fly.

But sometimes people can spend a lot of time and energy being angry about something, only to realize later on that it really didn't matter that much. When it comes to that kind of annoyance, it may be good to consider not getting angry in the first place.

Even if some situations have made you angry in the past, you may now choose not to let them bother you.

It might sound like I'm contradicting the previous chapter, but both ideas are true. Sometimes you can choose to get angry, and other times you can decide not to sweat the small stuff—and many of the things that can make a person angry might qualify as small stuff.

When it comes to irritations in everyday life, you can decide to just let them go. That might include situations like these:

- You take out your phone to make a call, only to find that the battery has run out.

- You're driving on a street where the speed limit is 40, and you end up behind a driver who's going 25 miles an hour.

- You've planned an afternoon picnic in the park, but a storm that wasn't in the forecast starts pouring rain with no letup in sight.

- You stop by the grocery store to pick up a couple of items you really need, and the person ahead of you in the express checkout didn't read—or chose to ignore—the "12 items or fewer" sign.

In instances like these, you might get angry and spend a lot of energy being upset, or you might choose to let go of the feelings that are building up, move past the incident as best you can, and not allow anger to take over.

Of course, "Don't sweat the small stuff" may sometimes be more easily said than done. Cancer is so stressful that your sensitivity to small stuff can be heightened. But even if you find yourself feeling angry for a moment, you may be able to take a deep breath, let it go, and choose not to let it consume you. Or, if you need to, take a little time for fast and furious venting, perhaps with a loved one or a trusted friend. But then, after you get it out of your system, move on instead of letting it ruin your day. A cancer survivor said, "One of the biggest things I learned from cancer is that it's up to *me* how I respond to any given situation."

Now, this doesn't mean that people should be hard on themselves if they do get angry. Sometimes fear and frustration build up, and the anger may flow before people have a chance to think about it. Later, they may look back and ask themselves, "Why did I waste energy getting upset about that?" If this happens, go easy on yourself. You're dealing with cancer, so you can cut yourself some slack.

When something irritates you, you can step back and ask yourself, "Is this really important? Will I even care about it tomorrow?" If the answer is "yes," you may want to get angry. But if the situation just doesn't matter much, you may choose to ignore it. A survivor said, "When I found myself getting angry about something minor, I'd just ask myself, 'Am I *really* going to let this bug me?' Then I'd recognize that it wasn't that big an issue and just laugh at the situation." Another person said, "I'd think, *If this is the worst thing that happens to me today, it will be a beautiful day.* That would put the annoyance in its place."

You are the only one who can decide what qualifies as *small stuff* for you. Then, when that small stuff threatens to make you angry, you actually may be happier if you choose not to sweat it.

Part 3

Becoming Informed

12

The Value of
Being Informed

*"The more you know and understand about
what's going on inside your body, the better
you'll be able to work with your medical team."*

Sometimes choices about cancer treatment may be crystal clear. Other times they can be as clear as mud.

This combination of clarity and uncertainty is why oncology, the study and treatment of cancer, is both a science and an art.

Science looks for demonstrated results that can be predictably repeated. Many aspects of cancer treatment fit that description. For example, if you have a particular type of tumor, scientific evidence may show that it's best to remove it surgically.

But cancer treatment choices aren't always that straightforward. With certain diagnoses, for instance, there may be two or more possible treatment options, each with its own advantages and disadvantages. If that's the situation, you and your loved ones will need to work with your oncologist and others on your medical team to decide on a course of treatment. Choices like these are where the art of treating cancer comes in—where medical professionals draw on their training, their experience, their unique perspective, and the patient's preferences as they weigh the options.

You'll work with your medical team to make decisions throughout treatment—some choices may be very clear, others less so. The more you learn about the cancer, the better you'll be able to participate in decision making and the more confident you'll be in your decisions. The rest of the chapters in part 3 can help with this process.

A survivor said, "You can't make good decisions without good information, so gather as much knowledge as you're able. Ask a lot of questions. Listen to informed opinions. Knowledge increases your power, decreases your fear, and gives you hope!"

13

Medical Questions to Ask and When to Ask Them

"When I was first diagnosed, my wife and I were in shock. We had no idea what questions we should ask about the surgery or the proposed treatment. We didn't even know how to spell the name of the cancer I had."

After you receive the news of the diagnosis, along with some initial information, the doctor invites you to ask any questions you may have. If you're like many people, this may be where you draw a blank. The news can be so overwhelming that you don't even know where to start.

That moment won't be your only chance to ask questions, though. You'll have more opportunities, not only at your next appointment but throughout treatment.

The purpose of this chapter is to give you ideas for questions you can ask at different times to get the information you need when you need it.

I've drawn the questions in this chapter from my own experience as well as the recommendations and experiences of a variety of medical professionals, survivors, and loved ones. You probably won't need to ask all the questions listed here, but I wanted to be as thorough as possible with these suggestions. They might also give you ideas for other questions.

Go Ahead and Ask Questions

Asking questions is a key to understanding and participating in your medical care. In fact, your medical team will welcome the questions you ask. Your questions are the best way to let them know what you're uncertain about and what you want to learn. As one cancer survivor put it, "My oncologist told me she wouldn't know what I was thinking or feeling unless I told her. She encouraged me to *ask anything* and *share everything.*"

An oncology nurse said, "I tell all our patients, 'There are no wrong questions, and your questions are never a bother. So ask away—we want you to get the answers you need.'"

Write a List of Questions

It can be helpful to write your list of questions and bring it to your appointment. When I did this, I left space between questions so I had room to take notes on the answers.

Bring Someone Along

It's beneficial to have someone with you at appointments to take notes, help you ask questions, and support you. Chapter 27, "Bring Someone with You to Appointments," chapter 28, "Take Notes," and chapter 29, "Focus Your Questions," include specific ways others can help you get the most from your appointments.

Questions to Ask

This chapter suggests possible questions to ask the physicians who work with you. The questions are grouped in the following categories:

I. **Questions to Ask Your Surgeon**

II. **Questions to Ask Your Oncologist about the Cancer's Type and Stage**

III. **Questions to Ask Your Oncologist about Tests, Imaging, or Procedures**

IV. **Questions to Ask Your Oncologist about Treatment Options**

V. **Questions to Ask Your Oncologist about Treatment Side Effects**

The purpose of these lists of questions is to save you time and effort. Reviewing these questions, possibly with a family member or close friend, can help you decide what to ask and might give you ideas for other questions.

Keep in mind that you won't need to ask all the questions listed because:

- Some of them might not apply to your situation.

- Your oncologist and others on your medical team will probably answer many of them before you ask.

- Your medical team may give you materials that address a number of questions.

- You may find answers to some of the questions as you do your own research (see chapter 14, "Where to Look for Information about Your Kind of Cancer").

Look at the information you already have, and then determine what questions you need to ask to fill in any gaps.

Since everyone's situation is unique, the order in which you ask questions may not be the same as the order in which they appear in this chapter. Also, you might address some of these questions to a nurse, a physician other than a surgeon or oncologist involved in your treatment, or another member of the medical team.

I. Questions to Ask Your Surgeon

Your cancer treatment may include surgery. If so, consider asking your surgeon some of the following questions.

Questions to Ask before Your Surgery

1. **What is the purpose or goal of this surgery?**

2. **What would be the likely outcome if I didn't have this surgery? Are there other options?**

3. **How soon should I have this surgery? What might be the risk in delaying it?**

4. **What will the surgery involve?**

5. **What are the risks associated with having this surgery? How likely are they to occur?**

6. **What role will pathology have during the surgery?**

    Sometimes during surgery, the surgeon will send a small sample of tissue to a pathologist to be examined right away. The pathologist's report will identify whether the tissue is cancerous. Pathologists also look at tissue samples after the surgery to make a more precise diagnosis.

7. **How long is the surgery likely to take?**

8. **What physical changes might I experience as a result of the surgery?**

9. **What's my expected overall recovery time?**

10. **What restrictions might there be on my activities after the surgery?**

11. **What type of assistance might I need during my recovery period?**

12. **When will I learn what you found during the surgery?**

Questions to Ask after Your Surgery

Here are some questions you could ask your surgeon in order to learn what was found during the surgery and what the findings mean.

1. **What was the outcome of the surgery? What did you find? Did you encounter anything unexpected?**

2. **Were there any complications? If so, how might they affect me?**

3. **Whom should I call if I have problems after office hours?**

4. **What activities should I avoid, and for how long?**

5. **When might it be possible to resume normal activities?**

    Explain to the surgeon what your normal activities are.

6. **What lifestyle changes, if any, could I make to help my recovery—for instance, changing my diet or doing special exercises?**

7. Would any specific therapy be helpful for me during recovery?

For example, physical therapy can help patients whose range of motion is limited due to their cancer or surgery, and speech therapy can help those who have problems with swallowing.

II. Questions to Ask Your Oncologist about the Cancer's Type and Stage

Once the pathology report or other test results come in, you'll talk with your oncologist about the type and stage of the cancer.

1. What is the specific type and stage of my cancer?

You probably already know the kind of cancer you're dealing with, but you may not be aware of its precise classification. Ask your oncologist to spell the name of the specific type of cancer—you'll need the correct spelling as you look for more information about it.

Knowing the stage of the cancer is also important. For most cancers, the stage is identified using the TNM system, which includes three different ratings:

T: The size and extent of the primary *tumor*

N: Whether the cancer has spread to lymph *nodes*

M: Whether the cancer has spread, or *metastasized,* to other parts of the body

Physicians will often combine the three ratings to determine an overall stage, indicated with a Roman numeral from I to IV and sometimes a letter as well. Certain cancers also have a stage 0, where the cancer has not spread to nearby tissues. The higher the stage number, the more advanced the cancer.

Some types of cancer use different systems. You may need to ask your oncologist to explain the system being used and what it means.

Staging is a major determining factor for treatment; different stages of the same cancer are often treated in different ways. Knowing the stage of the cancer will help you understand your treatment options.

2. How was the cancer's stage determined?

3. Has the cancer spread? If so, where has it spread?

4. How will my treatment be affected by the fact that the cancer has or hasn't spread?

5. How are we going to keep track of future cancer growth, if any occurs?

6. What are my treatment options? What would be the likely outcome, benefits, and risks of each option?

III. Questions to Ask Your Oncologist about Tests, Imaging, or Procedures

Your oncologist may order tests (such as a blood test), imaging (such as a CT scan, PET scan, or MRI), or procedures (such as a biopsy) to learn more about the cancer. The following questions can help you understand more about them.

1. What are the reasons for doing this [test, imaging, or procedure]? What could it tell us?

2. How is it done? How long will it take? Will it be uncomfortable?

3. Where is it done? Will it involve a hospital stay, or will it be done on an outpatient basis? Should I have someone provide transportation?

4. What are the benefits of having it done? What are the risks?

5. What should I do to prepare?

6. How and when will I find out the results and what they mean?

   Knowing approximately when you can expect the results can ease some of the anxiety during the wait.

7. Will I need to have it again? If so, when and how often?

IV. Questions to Ask Your Oncologist about Treatment Options

Asking questions such as these can help you understand your treatment options and make informed decisions.

1. What is the most frequently recommended treatment or treatments for this kind of cancer at this stage with these characteristics?

2. What treatment do you recommend? Why do you think that treatment is preferable for me?

> Every patient is unique, and your oncologist will consider many factors when recommending a treatment or combination of treatments. Make sure you understand the reasons for the recommendation. You will want to know how the treatment will help and what impact it may have on your day-to-day life.
>
> Sometimes an oncologist will present a patient with two or more treatment options to choose from. If that's your situation, ask for the information you need to understand each option and make a well-informed choice.

3. What is the treatment plan?

> For each treatment you consider, you'll want to discuss the schedule and related details.

- **How often will I receive the treatment?**
  Learn the treatment frequency—for example, it might take place once a day, once a week, once every three weeks, three weeks out of four, or on some other schedule.

- **How long will each individual treatment take?**

- **How long will the whole course of treatment last?**
  Keep in mind that the overall timeline for treatment may be adjusted later.

- **How will the treatment be given?**
  The treatment might be given orally, intravenously, by injection, through radiation, by other means, or by a combination of means.

- **Where will the treatment be given?**
  For many types of treatment, you'll go to a hospital or clinic as an outpatient. Depending upon your situation, you might take certain treatments at home, such as an oral medication or an intravenous medication using an infusion pump.

- **What are the names of the medications I'll be taking?**
  Write these down. Clarify the pronunciation and spelling so you can use them correctly in any future conversations or research. Your oncologist may give you articles or brochures about some medications.

- **Should I have someone come with me to treatment? Should I have someone provide transportation?**

4. **Will there be any other medical professionals involved in this treatment plan?**

   These may be current members of your medical team or people you haven't met yet, including a different type of oncologist (such as a radiation oncologist), a physician in another specialty, or other professionals who provide specific treatments.

5. **How will we know whether the treatment is working?**

   Find out what your team will use to monitor the effectiveness of the treatment and how frequently it will be used. These measures may include specific blood tests, CT scans, PET scans, MRIs, or other methods.

6. **What clinical trials might be appropriate for me?**

   Your oncologist may be aware of some clinical trial possibilities, or your own research might turn up options to discuss with him or her. Chapter 20, "Clinical Trials," says more about this.

7. **How soon should I start treatment? What might happen if I wait?**

   In some situations, it's vital to start treatment as soon as possible. For others, treatment doesn't need to begin immediately. If the need isn't urgent, you will have more time to consider the options, learn more, or get a second opinion before you begin treatment.

8. How might this treatment affect my day-to-day life?

Find out whether treatment will affect your ability to drive, work, or engage in other activities. Also ask whether you'll need to limit your contact with others for any reason.

9. How might this treatment affect my fertility? What are my options for having a child in the future?

10. Will I need to have any tests, imaging, or procedures before or during the course of treatment?

A blood test might be required before a treatment, for instance, to determine whether your white or red blood cell count or platelet count is sufficient for the treatment to take place. The physician may use a blood test to check the level of a tumor marker—a substance that can indicate the presence and extent of cancer—as a way of monitoring the effectiveness of the treatment. If you require a test, image, or procedure, see section III in this chapter, "Questions to Ask Your Oncologist about Tests, Imaging, or Procedures."

11. Is it okay to take my other medications or supplements?

Specify what your other medications and supplements are, including over-the-counter medications, and what dosages you take of each.

12. Are there certain foods I should avoid?

There may be substances within various foods that could interact unfavorably with a treatment medication, or there may be foods that typically don't agree with patients in a particular treatment regimen.

13. What lifestyle changes—for example, diet or special exercises—could I make to enhance the effectiveness of this treatment or decrease its side effects?

14. Are there certain activities I should limit or stop during this treatment?

V. Questions to Ask Your Oncologist about Treatment Side Effects

The following questions can help you find out what to expect and how best to deal with possible side effects (see chapter 22, "Side Effects").

1. **What are the possible side effects of this treatment? How likely are they to occur?**

2. **What medications or other means can be used to prevent, lessen, or manage expected side effects?**

3. **Do these medications for treating side effects have their own side effects? If so, what are they? How can I deal with them?**

   For example, a particular chemotherapy medication might have the side effect of nausea. There may be a medication that prevents or reduces the nausea but commonly has a side effect of constipation. You'd need to know this so you can plan to manage the constipation, perhaps through other medications or through your diet.

4. **Whom should I call if I start experiencing any side effects or have additional questions about side effects?**

5. **Whom should I call if I need to talk with someone after office hours?**

Giving careful thought to your questions will help you get the answers you need and make the most of your time with your medical team.

14

Where to Look for Information about Your Kind of Cancer

"For me, it was important to understand what was happening in my body and to educate myself about treatment options. The more I knew, the less afraid I was."

Learning about your kind of cancer can equip you and your loved ones to participate in the decisions ahead of you. This chapter describes places you might look in order to learn more about your kind of cancer. The goal is to help you gather accurate, reliable, up-to-date information efficiently and effectively by going to the best potential sources of knowledge, thus making the best use of your time.

Get Help If You Need It

The wide range of information sources in this chapter may seem like a lot to absorb, and the physical and emotional toll of cancer can sometimes leave you with little energy to do research. If that's the case, by all means ask others for assistance.

One survivor told me, "I knew from my own cancer experience how much misleading and unverified information is out there, especially on the internet. So when my dad was diagnosed, I offered to do all the information gathering for him. That way I could filter out everything except the most helpful, reliable, applicable material." A woman noted that she enlisted her daughter to help with her online research: "I felt completely helpless online, so knowing she would do that for me took a load off my mind."

Having the chance to help in this way may be deeply meaningful for your loved ones as well. A man whose wife had breast cancer told me, "Doing research gave me one more way to be actively involved in her care. It was something concrete I could do to be a big help to her." The sister of a survivor said, "Finding helpful material for my brother was empowering for both of us. It was like I was providing him with armor for the battlefield."

Frequently Used Sources

Here are some frequently used sources where you can find good information about your kind of cancer and its treatment. You'll find more about each of these sources on the pages that follow.

- Your oncologist and medical team
- Cancer associations—for cancer in general or specific kinds of cancer
- Cancer-related websites
- Medical dictionaries
- Books
- Reference librarians
- Cancer information centers
- Medical libraries
- Newsletters
- Medical journals
- Conferences and workshops
- Online communities
- People who have personal experience

You don't need to explore every one of these sources; using just a few of them can yield a lot of helpful information. I've listed all these to give you a number of options so you can get the greatest benefit from your time spent doing research.

The first three sources in the list—your oncologist and medical team, cancer associations, and cancer-related websites—are great places to begin learning more about your kind of cancer. You may want to concentrate your efforts on these sources first. Then consult other information sources as needed.

Of course, before acting on anything your research turns up, check with your medical team (see chapter 30, "Share Streamlined Information," for ideas about how to share this material in ways that make the best use of time).

Your Oncologist and Medical Team

Your number-one resource is your oncologist and his or her team. They can get you off to a great start in your learning, helping you understand what you need to know about your kind of cancer, your treatment options, and what to expect. They can recommend sources of information, help you make sense of what you find, and evaluate the information you share with them.

General Cancer Associations

General cancer associations can be valuable sources of information, especially as you begin your research. They can provide printed material, websites, and phone consultation to answer questions about cancer in general, as well as specific kinds of cancer.

Two particularly helpful sources are the American Cancer Society and the National Cancer Institute. Both provide resources designed for people who aren't medical professionals, so the information is presented in an easy-to-understand way.

American Cancer Society

The American Cancer Society (ACS) offers 24-hour phone support at 800-227-2345, with consultants on hand to answer your questions and point you to the best places to learn more. On the ACS website, cancer.org, you'll find booklets, brochures, and other material you can read online, save on your computer, or print out to read and share with family members. You can also request many of these materials to be sent to you by mail.

National Cancer Institute

The National Cancer Institute (NCI) is a federally sponsored division of the National Institutes of Health. You can reach the NCI by phone at 800-422-6237 (800-4-CANCER), Monday through Friday, 8:00 A.M. to 8:00 P.M. Eastern Time.

The NCI's Cancer Information Service provides information and answers to cancer-related questions by phone, email, or online chat on its website, cancer.gov.

The website offers information about many different kinds of cancer, current treatment information, listings of clinical trials, and news stories. The NCI has a variety of booklets and brochures available online or by mail.

Specific Cancer Associations

In addition to general cancer associations, you may also find foundations, associations, and societies that focus on a specific kind of cancer—for example, the International Liver Cancer Association or the Leukemia and Lymphoma Society. Often, these associations provide reliable information through websites, newsletters, and links to other sources. Many have discussion groups where you can interact with others dealing with that kind of cancer. One survivor told me, "I've gotten really helpful information from the foundations that focus on my kind of cancer. They know about the latest research and treatment information, and they update regularly."

You can find these organizations by checking with your medical team or doing an online search. Using a search engine, type the name of your specific kind of cancer plus the word *foundation, association,* or *society.* The chances are good that you'll find a number of organizations worth checking out. If you're unsure about an organization's credibility, ask your medical team.

Cancer-Related Websites

The internet can be an excellent source for up-to-date, specific information about your kind of cancer and its treatment. Besides the American Cancer Society and National Cancer Institute websites, you can get valuable information from other reputable medical and cancer-related websites. Here are some examples:

- **NCCN.org/patients** is the patient page for the National Comprehensive Cancer Network, a nonprofit organization working to advance cancer research and treatment. The website includes a wide range of resources for patients and caregivers, including extensive guidelines for some of the most common kinds of cancer.

- **Cancer.net** is the patient information website of the American Society of Clinical Oncology. It offers information about many specific kinds of cancer, including symptoms, staging, treatment, clinical trials, side effects, and current research. An editorial board of more than 150 oncologists and other medical professionals regularly reviews the website's content.

- **PubMed,** a database of publications in the National Library of Medicine, is available at ncbi.nlm.nih.gov/pubmed. You can enter particular keywords, such as your specific kind of cancer or a medication name, into the search engine to find articles on the desired subject. Then, you can use various filters to narrow down the articles to those most helpful for you. Some articles are free; others are available for purchase. Many of these articles are technical in nature, so it can be helpful to have a medical dictionary as you read them.

- **MedlinePlus.gov** is the National Institutes of Health's website for patients and their loved ones. It provides information about diseases, conditions, and wellness issues. You'll find a medical dictionary, information about medications, a medical encyclopedia, names of organizations related to specific kinds of cancer, and other resources.

- **Medscape.com** provides news about a variety of medical areas, including oncology. You can register free of charge to get access to the articles and receive regular updates by email. Such updates are a good way to keep your knowledge current.

You can use an online search engine to find other websites—but be cautious about trusting what you find on the internet. Not all websites provide reliable information. Some website owners want to help you; others are out to take advantage of you. (See the section "How to Identify Accurate, Reliable Information on the Internet" later in this chapter.)

Most importantly, before you act on any information you find online, check with your oncologist or another member of your medical team to confirm its accuracy and its applicability to your situation.

Medical Dictionaries

As you dig into your research, you may start coming across potentially unfamiliar terms like *neuropathy, alopecia, edema,* or *immunotherapy.* You may need a medical dictionary to translate some of what you read. A family member of a survivor put it this way: "For me, cancer was like a trip to a foreign country—I needed to learn the language to get anywhere."

While you can find medical dictionaries in print, often a convenient option is to use an online medical dictionary. Here are two resources geared toward people who aren't medical professionals:

- The MedlinePlus website, which is operated by the National Institutes of Health, offers a general medical dictionary at medlineplus.gov/mplusdictionary.html.

- The National Cancer Institute website includes a cancer-specific online dictionary at cancer.gov/dictionary.

Being able to understand and use some medical terminology will help you communicate with your medical team more effectively and efficiently.

Books

In order to dig deeper, it may help to get one or more books about your kind of cancer. Such a book can give you a wealth of information in one place, helping you gain a broad understanding of your kind of cancer without having to consult numerous resources.

Determine whether you want a book written for medical professionals or the general public. When you're trying to learn about a specific kind of cancer, a book for professionals may have more extensive information, but it may also be harder to follow because of technical medical language. Some people find these books valuable as reference texts, reading the parts that are relevant to them with a medical dictionary at hand. Books written for a wider audience are usually easier to read and can vary in the scope of their content.

You could ask your medical team to suggest helpful books to read. They can recommend one or more to get you started.

You could also see what books are available by searching an online bookstore. Narrow your search to books on your specific kind of cancer.

Many cancer-related books are autobiographical in nature, focusing on the author's own story. While books like these are often inspiring and interesting to read, they may not provide as much specific information about dealing with cancer.

Reference Librarians

You may want to contact the reference librarian at your local library for help with finding information about your kind of cancer. Reference librarians are specially trained to find information about specific topics and evaluate print and online resources. People regularly call them to ask for help with their research. They can work with you to find articles, newsletters, reputable medical journals, associations for your specific kind of cancer, and other sources of useful information.

If your local library isn't able to provide the help you need, you might want to call a larger library and ask to speak with a reference librarian there. He or she may be able to assist you over the phone and send you documents or links by email.

Cancer Information Centers

A number of hospitals and treatment centers have a cancer information center. This is usually an area where you can find books, booklets, brochures, and other information about various kinds of cancer. If you need help, ask the cancer information center staff.

Medical Libraries

Some hospitals and medical centers have a medical library with cancer resources that patients and others may borrow. Ask a librarian to help you find resources about your kind of cancer. If your hospital doesn't have a cancer information center or medical library with cancer resources, you can ask your medical team about other places to look.

Another good place to do research is a university or medical school library. If you have such a school in your area, visit its library and ask a reference or research librarian for assistance.

Newsletters

Newsletters, in print and online, are available about many kinds of cancer. They may contain information about treatments, dates for conferences and workshops, tips on handling side effects, and much more.

Your medical team may be able to direct you to a newsletter for your kind of cancer. Another good way to find newsletters is by using an online search engine and searching for the name of your specific cancer plus the word *newsletter.*

Medical Journals

It can be helpful to find reputable medical or scientific journals that focus on particular kinds of cancer. These journals are written by medical professionals and other scientists for their peers and often include technical language, so you might focus more on other resources first. Still, you may be able to learn some good information about your kind of cancer if you read some relevant journal articles with a medical dictionary handy.

Similar to searching for newsletters, you can find journal websites by doing an online search for the name of a kind of cancer plus *journal.* You might also search for journal articles about particular kinds of cancer or other topics at the PubMed website, ncbi.nlm.nih.gov/pubmed. Often you can read abstracts that summarize articles, and sometimes you can access entire articles online.

Conferences and Workshops

As you gather information about your kind of cancer, you might find out about conferences and workshops that would be helpful for you. Such meetings can provide information about treatments or clinical trials and how you might benefit from them.

One reason to attend conferences in person is that they're great places for networking. You might meet people who are able to share useful information and support. If you can't attend in person, however, you may be able to view these events via live stream or download.

Online Communities

Here are three examples of online communities that can help you learn more about your kind of cancer:

- **Discussion Boards.** You can often find several online message boards, forums, or other groups for discussing your kind of cancer by doing an online search including the words *online discussion board, online message board,* or something similar, along with your kind of cancer. To join one of these groups, you'll probably have to register, typically free of charge.

- **Blogs.** Some people write blogs about cancer in general or their own personal cancer experiences. You can find many different blogs through an online search—as you do, evaluate them carefully to determine which ones might meet your needs. Some share helpful information, but others may not be as applicable to your situation.

- **Social Media.** Social media can be a way to get in touch with cancer-related groups or others in your situation. Search social media sites or services using the name of your kind of cancer, and you will likely find one or more groups to join or follow.

Be careful about information you find via online communities—it may sometimes be based more on opinion than on fact. If you read about a promising new clinical trial or other information that catches your eye, find out what you can about it and then talk with your oncologist or another member of your medical team about its accuracy and applicability to your situation.

People Who Have Personal Experience

Finally, you can also learn a lot from people who have personal experience with your kind of cancer. See chapter 15, "Network with People Who Have Been There."

How to Identify Accurate, Reliable Information on the Internet

The internet is a great source of information, but it's a little like the Wild West—a vast frontier with amazing resources and tremendous potential, yet untamed, unregulated, and downright dangerous at times. You can find a lot of cancer-related information on the internet, but not all of it will be helpful or even reliable—and misinformation lurks there as well.

Here are a number of filters to help you sift through information on the internet and determine what is likely to be reliable and accurate:

1. **Author.** Look for who wrote or developed the material. If it's a medical school or organization, a cancer society, or someone with an M.D. or a Ph.D., that's usually a good initial sign.

2. **Web Address.** A web address ending with .edu or .gov is more likely to be reliable. One ending in .com generally indicates a commercial website, which means it *might* contain information biased toward selling particular products or services. An address ending with .org generally indicates a not-for-profit organization. Some nonprofits, like the American Cancer Society (cancer.org), are well known and highly respected; with others, you may need to learn more about the organization before deciding what to do with the information.

3. **Date.** Find the date or the copyright on the webpage to learn when the information was most recently revised. The more current the information, the more reliable it's likely to be. If there's no date, it's harder to be sure how current and reliable the information is.

4. **About Us.** Most websites have an "About Us" page that tells about the sponsor of the website, whether it's an organization or one or more individuals. Check that page out and ask yourself questions such as: *What is the mission of this website and its sponsor? What are the sponsor's core values—stated or implied? How well known and respected is the sponsor? What is this website trying to accomplish, and is it in my best interests?*

5. **Facts.** Look for websites containing factual information rather than personal opinions. A site that is heavy on individual testimonials about a specific treatment and light on facts is probably less reliable. Also check whether the information is documented with statistics, studies, or articles from sources you know are reliable. The website is more likely to be trustworthy if it cites studies published in reputable medical or scientific journals.

If a website touts personal testimonies from people who claim to have been cured or otherwise benefited from a treatment, make sure the claims are backed up by scientifically sound studies. Individual success stories can be misleading, as there can be many reasons why a cancer patient's condition improves. A scientifically valid study, however, can determine whether a particular treatment actually caused any benefits.

6. **Links.** Does the website include any links to reputable websites such as those maintained by cancer associations, medical schools, or physician organizations? If so, the content is more likely to be reliable.

7. **Ads.** If the website contains ads promoting products or services, some of the information on that website could be biased toward those items.

8. **Where Else the Information Appears.** Check other sources to see whether they agree with the information provided by the website. The more places the information can be found—especially if some of those are print rather than online resources—the more likely that information is accurate.

9. **What Your Oncologist Thinks of the Information.** The best way for you to check the reliability of what you learn on the internet is to ask your oncologist about it. See chapter 30, "Share Streamlined Information," for how to share your research with the medical team.

The Goal: Seek Out the Best

Whether you do the research yourself or have someone else lend a hand, your goal is to seek out the best, most accurate and complete information from the best, most reliable sources.

One survivor summed it up this way: "Having knowledge reduced my fear. I needed to know what I was up against and what the options were so I could be part of choosing the best plan to defeat it."

15

Network with People Who Have Been There

"I was always on the lookout for people who were as determined to defeat their cancer as I was to defeat mine. People like that are great for exchanging insights and experiences with."

One way to quickly and effectively learn about your kind of cancer is by talking to people who have firsthand experience with it, whether they've had cancer or supported a loved one with cancer. I like to say these people are "P.H.D.s"—they have a ***Personal History with the Disease.*** They've been through a lot of the challenges, they've learned a great deal, and they've scouted ahead for pitfalls and opportunities. Although your oncologist and medical team will be your main source of information, these P.H.D.s can be an invaluable resource as well, and I've found that they're almost always glad to help.

One woman told me of the benefits of finding such a person: "Having someone to talk to—someone who had been there—was so helpful. Not only could she answer many of my questions, but just being face to face with someone who had made it through this ordeal worked wonders for my soul."

Keep in mind that other people's experiences won't perfectly mirror your own. There are varieties of each kind of cancer, and even if someone has the exact cancer and treatment that you have, your body's responses to the cancer and to the treatment might be different. Also be aware that not all those who have experience with cancer will share information that's helpful to you.

That being said, many of these P.H.D.s will share a lot of useful knowledge and resources with you, even if their cancer experience differs from yours—and maybe you can do the same for them.

Where to Find People Who Have Experience

P.H.D.s are out there, and you can find them with a little searching. Here are some good places to begin.

People You Already Know

Check with relatives, friends, neighbors, coworkers, or people in a congregation, club, or other group you're connected with. Tell them the kind of cancer you have, and let them know you're trying to find people who have experience with it. A neighbor might know someone who leads a cancer support group. Your coworker might have a friend who has dealt with the same kind of cancer.

You never know what kind of help you'll find until you ask. One man told me:

> "I made one of my best connections at the golf course. A friend introduced me to a man who had survived the same kind of cancer. He had all kinds of wisdom, experience, and encouragement to share and became a great source of help."

As one survivor put it:

> "Nowadays, it seems like everyone you meet has some connection to cancer. If you ask enough people for help, pretty soon someone will put you in touch with a person they know who has experienced your kind of cancer."

People You Meet during Treatment

Many people have told me they met some of the most helpful P.H.D.s in their oncologist's waiting room, in the chemotherapy treatment room, or at the radiation therapy center.

Once, when I was in the waiting area while Joan was undergoing an outpatient surgical procedure, I began talking with a man whose wife was going through a similar procedure. As we talked, I realized he had a great deal of insight and experience to share. We soon became great allies, discussing the challenging treatment decisions we and our wives faced. And this relationship, which began for the purpose of sharing information, developed into a long-lasting friendship.

Social Media

Some people have said they've found P.H.D.s through social media. A good way to start is by posting a carefully written note like this:

> I've just been diagnosed with [kind of cancer], and I want to learn more about it. I'd like to talk with anyone who could share about his or her experience with [kind of cancer].

Anyone—a college student or a grandmother, a patient or a family member—could respond to you. People have told me they've made connections with others all over the world. Of course, you'll need to be careful about information and connections you find online—not everything or everyone will be reliable or helpful for you.

Local Support Groups

Hospitals, cancer treatment centers, cancer-related associations, congregations, and other organizations in your community may offer support groups for people with specific kinds of cancer and for their families. Your oncologist may have information about support groups in your area.

In addition to offering you the opportunity to share your thoughts and feelings, these support groups can be a good place to learn about others' experiences and what they've found helpful. Here's what a survivor said: "My cancer support group was amazing. With the experiences shared, answers to questions, stories, camaraderie, prayers, and hope, I never felt alone on this journey." See chapter 65, "Consider a Support Group," for more information.

Conferences and Workshops

As noted in chapter 14, "Where to Look for Information about Your Kind of Cancer," conferences and workshops about your specific kind of cancer are often great places to meet people going through an experience much like yours. At one such conference I met a man whose wife's cancer was similar to Joan's. Although he lived across the country from me, we regularly kept in touch by email and phone, sharing information we learned. We were able to help each other with research and support each other through the highs and lows we experienced.

Local Cancer Awareness Activities

Many communities and hospitals hold cancer awareness events, rallies, runs, dinners, or fundraisers. Some are specific to certain kinds of cancer; others are more general. All of them give you opportunities to meet

P.H.D.s—including survivors, family members of people with cancer, and other supporters who are passionate about defeating cancer and eager to help others.

The wife of a man with cancer said, "We met many survivors through the American Cancer Society Relay for Life in our community. The organizer of the local Relay was farther along in treatment than my husband, and he was amazingly open in sharing information and feelings."

Getting Connected through a Cancer Association

Many cancer associations will help you reach others who have the same kind of cancer as you. One cancer survivor said, "Not only did they connect me by phone with people who had my form of cancer, but they also hosted webinars with treatment specialists. They were an excellent resource!" Chapter 14 talks about how you can find an association for your kind of cancer.

Asking Your Hospital or Cancer Center to Match You with Someone

Many hospitals and cancer centers have programs that will connect you with someone who has experienced your kind of cancer. If no such program is available in your area, contact the Cancer Hope Network—its website is cancerhopenetwork.org. This organization provides free, confidential support by matching patients with trained volunteers who've had a similar cancer experience.

Internet Groups

During Joan's fight against cancer, a friend told us about an online ovarian cancer discussion group. We checked out the website, joined the discussion group, and found some useful information from others who had experienced what we were going through. Chapter 14 gives some ideas about how to find online discussion boards, forums, and other groups for sharing information about your kind of cancer.

What to Ask

Here are some basic questions you might ask when talking with P.H.D.s:

- "What do you know now that you wish you had known earlier?"

- "What websites, social media, or internet groups have you found most valuable? Which ones weren't helpful?"

- "What books, pamphlets, or other materials did you find helpful?"

- "What support groups have you found to be helpful?"

- "After treatment, what was the recovery process like?"

- "What lifestyle changes or limitations did you and your family experience during or after treatment?"

- "What side effects did you or your loved one experience? What helpful ideas did you learn for minimizing or managing them?"

- "Did you or your loved one need to make any dietary changes? What changes did you find helpful?"

- "Do you know anyone else who has experience with this kind of cancer?"

- "What else should I know?"

Use this list as a starting point and ask other questions as they come up.

Contacting People You've Never Met

As you search for people to network with, you may come across the names of people you've never met who seem like potential allies. Maybe a friend gave you the name of a cousin who had your kind of cancer, or perhaps you read about a survivor in a newspaper or online article. In situations like these, you may wonder whether to contact a complete stranger out of the blue.

I encourage you to go ahead and reach out to the person. I've found that people who have experience with cancer are typically open to sharing information with others. When you are courteous, warm, and respectful, you will usually be met with the same attitude. And if the person can't help in the way you need, he or she may direct you to someone else who can. One person told me:

> "One of my most valuable contacts was someone I'd never even met face to face—a long-distance friend of a friend who had survived the same kind of cancer I had. I went ahead and called her one day, and she was glad to help me. We had a great conversation. I believe she's part of the reason I'm alive today, and I'm grateful to her."

Run Ideas Past Your Medical Team

When your networking provides information you think might help, talk about it with your medical team. Your team will be able to evaluate the information and let you know how reliable and potentially useful it is.

Invaluable Allies

One woman described her P.H.D. friend like this:

> "She was around my own age, had been through a similar cancer, and was eager to help. We met through a mutual friend and talked at least once a week. She knew the ropes, could give me an idea of what to expect, and was filled with practical tips on everything. She made all the difference in the world to me."

As you learn about your kind of cancer, you don't have to try to do everything by yourself. People who've already faced the challenges you're experiencing can be invaluable allies. You can learn from what they've found out, build on information they've gathered, and gain insights from what they've experienced.

16

Keeping Track of Personal Medical Information

"Right after my diagnosis, my daughter gave me a bright purple notebook. I kept all my medical information in there—I could just pick it up to check something or take it with me to appointments. Everything I needed was in that notebook."

Over the course of your fight with cancer, you can end up with a lot of medical and treatment information, including:

- your own notes;
- test results;
- treatment schedules;
- X-rays, CT scans, and other images;
- information about medications; and
- other medical reports and records.

Keeping track of this information will ensure that it's easily accessible when you need it.

The purpose of this chapter is to share some possibilities for what medical information you might want to save and ways to keep track of it.

Ask for Help

As you read this chapter, you might think, *This sounds good to do, but I'm not the best at organization,* or *I don't know how I'd find the time and energy to do this right now.* Some people find this kind of organizing easy, but for others, the thought of it makes their head swim.

This isn't something you have to do alone, though. You can enlist the help of family members or friends, possibly showing them this chapter to give them ideas about what to do. One person said:

> "My mother tracked everything for me. She kept an accordion file that had different folders for my tests, meds, surgeries, visits, questions, and so on, and we brought it along to every appointment. It was helpful to have all the information right at our fingertips. She told me, 'This is something I can do to help you.'"

Reasons for Keeping Track of Your Medical Information

Having a record of your medical and treatment history can simplify things for you in a number of ways:

- Keeping track of medical information lets you go back over your treatment history if you're not sure about something. A survivor said, "I saved everything I could. With all the stress of treatment, I couldn't always remember everything, so it was good to be able to check back just to verify something I thought I remembered."

- If you get a second opinion or consult with another specialist, you'll want to bring along your medical information to provide details about what's happened so far in your treatment.

- If you apply for a clinical trial, you'll need to give the coordinator up-to-date information about your diagnosis and treatment history.

- Bringing key medical information with you to appointments can save a lot of time for you and your medical team. One man said, "Having my medical information with me helped me quickly answer the doctor's questions and give an accurate picture of what was going on."

- Keeping track of personal medical information is a way to show your medical team that you want to be an active partner in your treatment. One person told me, "My doctor visits were more productive because I kept everything so organized. The doctors appreciated how I kept track of treatments, medications, and my own condition from visit to visit."

Here's another important reason: Managing the information about your medical and treatment history can give you a sense of control at a time when your world has been turned upside down. A survivor said, "Since I had all my information in one place, *I felt in control.* Whenever I wanted to, I could go back and find exactly what I needed to remember. It was very empowering."

Some Thoughts about Electronic and Printed Medical Records

If you have online access to your medical records, find out what information is available to you and how to retrieve it. If you don't have access to the records you need, you might request printed copies of various reports so you can personally review them.

In addition, find out who on your medical team has access to your electronic medical records and what, if anything, you need to do to give your other physicians access to the specific information they need.

Even if you and all the medical professionals you're working with have access to your electronic records, it can still be helpful for you to keep printed copies. At some point, you may see a new physician who doesn't yet have access to your electronic records, or you may not be able to retrieve a report electronically right away. Having printed copies can help in these situations.

What Personal Medical Information to Keep

You may want to keep diagnosis and treatment information like the following.

Your own notes. This includes any notes taken by you or someone who comes with you to medical appointments.

Addresses and phone numbers for physicians' offices, hospitals, and other facilities. A clear plastic sleeve that holds business cards can be helpful for keeping contact information readily available, especially if you store your personal medical information in a notebook or file folders. You also might keep the information in your contact list on a mobile device or computer.

A chronological summary of your diagnosis and treatments. Joan and I created a summary of all her diagnoses, treatments, tests, and procedures in the order she had them, and we updated it after every appointment, test, or treatment. See the appendix, "Chronological Diagnosis and Treatment Tracking Tools," which describes what you might include in such a summary and presents a fictional example.

A calendar record of your diagnosis and treatments. Joan and I also created a series of calendar pages that showed the dates of past treatments, tests of tumor marker levels, scans and other images, office visits, surgeries, and other tests or procedures. The appendix gives ideas for information to include in calendar pages like these, along with a fictional example.

Test results, pathology reports, and operative reports. You can obtain copies of test results and reports after each biopsy, medical test, or surgical procedure.

Imaging reports such as X-rays, CT or PET scans, and MRIs. You can get copies of imaging reports as well as digital copies of the actual images.

Tumor marker levels. Some cancers have specific markers found in the blood. The level of these markers can indicate the cancer's activity.

Current medications, dosages, and schedules. You can keep a list of all medications you take—not only prescription medications but also over-the-counter items. Include the dosage amounts and dosage schedules. Also keep a record of any medications that you are allergic to or that you otherwise cannot tolerate, along with the specific effects they have.

A dietary log. A registered dietitian or other member of your medical team may provide dietary guidance and suggest that you keep a dietary log. Knowing what foods you can and can't tolerate and what effects they have will assist your team in designing a nutrition plan that works for you.

A personal log or side-effects log. Many cancer patients say they benefit from keeping a record of how they feel each day during treatment. This may be a calendar with brief notes to keep track of symptoms and side effects. (See chapter 22, "Side Effects," for more ideas on putting together a log specifically for side effects.) A log like this can be a source of personal reassurance. A person with lymphoma told me, "I could look back at my log and see that I usually felt sick on the third day after treatment, but that the symptoms went away by the fourth or fifth day. That gave me encouragement and strength to carry on."

A pain journal. Some cancer patients work with their medical team to develop a pain management plan, which may include a pain journal where patients record their level of pain on a regular basis. (See chapter 21, "Pain Management.")

A calendar of upcoming appointments and other key dates. Some find it helpful to set up a calendar of upcoming appointments, treatments, tests, and procedures. You can include any instructions you receive about what to do (such as taking preparatory medications) or not to do (such as not eating certain foods) prior to specific treatments, tests, or procedures.

Questions. No doubt you'll have questions over the course of treatment, as will those close to you. As you or your loved ones think of questions, write them down. Then, when you prepare for an appointment, you can choose the questions that are most appropriate for that visit. (See chapter 13, "Medical Questions to Ask and When to Ask Them," and chapter 29, "Focus Your Questions.")

This can be a lot of information to keep track of. I'm including all these ideas to give you options. You can pick and choose which ones feel right to you—or include other information you think you'll need.

How to Organize Your Personal Medical Information

Two keys to organizing your medical information are to:

1. keep it as simple as possible; and

2. make it easy to locate specific items.

Here are a few ideas about how to do that.

On a Computer or Other Electronic Device

Some people choose to store personal medical information electronically.

- You could scan notes and reports into your computer.

- You might use a camera or mobile device to take photos—perhaps of prescription labels, of documents, or of physical changes you want to keep track of—and then store the photos on your computer.

- You might store images and information on a tablet or laptop computer.

A survivor told me:

"I kept a spreadsheet to track doctors' appointments, tests, and notes—creating a separate page for each doctor or hospital. I also scanned records and reports so I could store and organize them digitally, and I used a couple of smartphone apps to help track how my body was doing. I found it much easier to find what I needed that way, and it helped me to pull a variety of documents together into a simple system."

Remember that it may not be convenient to show medical team members a document on a small screen. Also, you may need printed copies of documents if you want to pass them along.

In File Folders

Other people feel more comfortable working with paper and file folders. One survivor said, "Even though I kept information on my laptop, I also liked having physical copies of certain items in file folders. It feels like the information is real when I can hold the pages in my hands."

There are advantages to keeping information in file folders.

- Many of your records and reports will be on paper and can easily be stored this way.

- It's easy to add and reorganize material as you gather information.

You might keep the file folders in a plastic file box or accordion file with a divider for each type of information.

In a Three-Ring Binder

Still another option is to store your medical records in a three-ring binder. You can create sections in the binder for different kinds of information and then make a tab for each section. After each appointment, you can add the latest material to the appropriate sections.

You might organize the information in each section in reverse chronological order—the oldest information in the back of the section and the newest in front. This method can give you a clear picture of everything from the time of diagnosis up to the most recent updates.

A woman talked about how well this worked for her father:

"Dad has always been a methodical record keeper, so right after his diagnosis he set up a three-ring binder. At the time, I didn't realize how much of a help it would be. But as the list of team members grew, along with all the tests, treatments, and everything else, keeping everything organized in one place saved us a lot of time and stress."

Tell Someone How You've Organized Your Information

Make sure to tell one or more people how you've organized your information and how to access it. That way, if you need something but aren't able to get to it, such as during a hospital stay, you can ask someone to retrieve it for you.

Having your personal medical information available and easy to find can be a great help. The ideas in this chapter describe some possibilities—use the approach that works best for you.

17

Thanking People Who Have Helped You Learn More

"It's healing to say 'thank you' to people who've helped you out. An expression of thanks is a gift of grace."

It's always good to thank people for *any* kind of help they give you. But it's especially important to express gratitude to people who share helpful information. Although thanking people may come naturally to us under most circumstances, it can easily fall by the wayside in the midst of everything connected to cancer, so it's worth some extra attention.

Thanking people who've taken time to share information with you is a good idea for a couple of reasons:

- First, it lets people know that you genuinely value them and appreciate their sharing and insights. It shows them how much of a difference they've made for you. One person who has helped many cancer patients learn more said, "Everyone likes to be appreciated. When others thank me, I feel valued and affirmed, and I know I've been of service—I can see I've left my mark. Hearing someone say 'thank you' shows me that I matter and that my efforts are worth it."

- Second, by letting others know that you are truly grateful for their assistance, you're strengthening your relationship with people who genuinely want to help you. They'll often be glad to help again if you need it later on. One person with cancer said, "A 'thank you' completes the circle by letting people know that their helping hand was welcomed and appreciated. Sometimes they need that connection in order to feel free to continue helping." Another person told me, "I'm always willing to go the second mile when someone has said 'thank you' for the first mile."

Some Ways to Say Thank You

Of course, people appreciate it when you thank them at the time they share information with you.

After that, you might want to send a short thank-you note. A note from the heart is a powerful way to let someone know how much you value him or her.

If possible, you might consider writing the message by hand to make your thank-you even more personal. A *Wall Street Journal* article described the meaning found in a handwritten note:

> Handwriting . . . forms a direct and intimate bridge between two people. We know, deep down, that there's nothing to match the communication with a pen on paper, and we tend to connect this feeling with our highest intentions.[1]

Keep your thank-you simple. It isn't necessary to write a lot—a brief note that gets right to the point is enough to express your appreciation.

If you don't feel up to sending a thank-you note right away, that's all right. You could ask a loved one or a friend to write the note for you, or you could wait and write one when you're better able to do so. If you decide to wait until you're feeling better, you can keep a list of the names of the people you want to be sure to thank later on.

Some people have told me they felt comfortable using email or social media to express their thanks, while others have said they prefer sending thank-yous by mail. If you aren't sure which method to use, I'd recommend sending a note or a card. A warm, personal thank-you in the mail is becoming increasingly rare, so yours will really stand out.

Additional Expressions of Gratitude

In some cases, you might want to go beyond spoken or written expressions of gratitude. If someone has helped you a great deal in your information-gathering or provided you with an extremely helpful bit of wisdom, you might give him or her a gift or some other token of your appreciation. For instance, one couple

---

1 Philip Hensher, "The Lost Art of the Handwritten Note," *Wall Street Journal,* December 29–30, 2012, p. C3.

had given Joan and me a lot of knowledge and support, so we took them to dinner one evening.

Here are a few ideas others have shared with me:

- A woman said, "When my treatments were all over, I took a bouquet of flowers to a woman who was a godsend when it came to helpful information."

- After one survivor's treatments were behind him and he regained his strength, he learned that a man who had provided him with some very helpful resources needed to go out of town for a weekend but had no one to watch his two dogs. The survivor volunteered to care for the man's pets as a way to thank him for his assistance.

- Other people told me they've given a fruit basket, movie tickets, a restaurant gift certificate, a bottle of wine, or another gift as an expression of gratitude.

When you take time to thank people for helping you obtain needed information, it warms their hearts as well as yours. It's a simple act that has a powerful effect.

18

Updating People Who Have Helped You Learn More

"When people helped me, that meant they cared about me, so I knew they really wanted to know what I did with their suggestions."

Have you ever shared useful information or helped a person think through a situation—and later heard back from the person saying something like, "You know that conversation we had last fall? Well, I did what we talked about, and it's worked out really well for me." It means a lot to learn that you helped make a difference for someone. Even if the person says, "I thought carefully about your suggestion, and here's what I did instead . . . ," it's still gratifying to know that he or she cares enough to keep you informed.

Updating people who have provided useful information about cancer can be gratifying for them in the same way.

In this chapter, I'm not talking about updating your family and friends. That topic will be addressed in chapter 54, "Keeping Family and Friends Up to Date." I'm talking about sharing updates with the same people as in chapter 17—those who have helped you learn more.

You've already thanked these people, but bringing them up to date later on tells them that you still value and appreciate their help. A woman who is frequently asked for advice about cancer told me, "When I've helped someone who has cancer, and then that person gives me an update, I take that as an expression of trust and confidence. It makes me feel like part of the person's team, and I feel really good about that."

Nurture Your Network

As people help you find information, you are building a network of support-ive individuals who have the ability or experience to help you in significant ways. Providing them with updates is a way of nurturing that network and keeping the lines of communication open. If you need to ask them for help again, they will be more likely to respond if you've shown them the courtesy of letting them know how things are going with you. Plus, your update may stimulate their thinking and bring to mind other ideas or suggestions they want to share with you.

One survivor said, "My wife and I learned a lot from some people who'd had cancer, and we kept in touch with them even after we moved out of town. Because we stayed connected to them and sent the occasional update, they ended up sharing several additional ideas that really helped us."

As Needed, Enlist Friends or Family to Help You Update People

Maybe you're thinking, *It's all I can do to keep up with my treatments. I don't have the time or energy to update people who have helped me.* This can be a great time to call on a friend or family member for help.

People in your life often appreciate having something specific they can do for you. A survivor told me, "My sister's help with updating people meant a lot to me, and it also benefited her to know she was helping me in a meaningful way."

It doesn't really matter if someone else provides the update on your behalf. What matters is that the person on the receiving end knows that you ap-preciate him or her.

Some Ideas about Updating People

Tailor your update to the situation. Sometimes a quick email or phone call is all it takes. Other times a short letter might work better—or, with someone who was especially helpful, maybe a face-to-face update.

Since these people have helped you, it's a good idea to personalize your communication rather than simply adding their names to your general email list or pointing them to a personal webpage. General email or webpage updates work well for sharing news with larger numbers of friends and extended family members at once (see chapter 54, "Keeping Family and Friends Up to Date," for more about such updates). With those who have gone out of their way to help you or whose help you may need again, however, a more individual approach is often preferable. It's better to communicate with those people directly and personally as you are able.

Often, a quick, to-the-point communication works best. You're busy, and the other person is too. Your message can simply:

- express your appreciation for the help the person has given you;

- tell how you're doing; and

- say how the information helped you.

Here's the text of a brief letter I wrote to a person who helped Joan and me along the way:

> *We wanted to let you know that Joan was able to get into the clinical trial you told us about. We asked her oncologist about it, and he thought it was a great idea. So he helped pave the way, and now she's in!*
>
> *Thank you for all your kind assistance over the past few months. Given the challenges we've been facing, being able to call and talk with you has been very helpful.*
>
> *By the way, on Father's Day we went to the restaurant you recommended. The food was as great as you said it would be.*

The letter was short but personal. In addition to telling how the person's help had made a difference, it conveyed friendly feelings and showed our gratitude for the person's help.

When to Update People

While you might send general updates to extended family and friends on a regular basis, you'll probably send less frequent updates to those who have helped you learn more.

You can include a short update in a thank-you note you send after the person helped you, as mentioned in chapter 17, "Thanking People Who Have Helped You Learn More." Later, you can update the person again if something happens that's related to the information he or she gave you—for example, if you read and benefited from an article the person told you about, or if you've been getting good results from a tip he or she gave you.

Why It's Important to Update People

Chapter 17 lists two important reasons for thanking people:

- It shows how much you value them.

- When people know that their assistance is welcomed and appreciated, it strengthens the relationship, and they are more likely to offer additional help in the future.

These reasons are just as true when it comes to updating people.

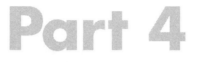

Part 4

Understanding Medical Matters

19

Getting a
Second Opinion

"After consulting with my oncologist about it, I decided to seek a second opinion. Getting input from another physician gave me greater peace of mind; I knew that I was making the best decision about my treatment."

Some people get a second opinion as part of learning about their diagnosis and treatment options. This chapter provides information to help you decide whether to seek a second opinion and describes how to go about getting one.

What a Second Opinion Is

After working with an oncologist or other physician who has made a diagnosis and proposed a treatment plan, a patient may choose to consult with a second physician, who will come to an independent conclusion about the diagnosis and recommend a course of treatment. This second opinion may:

- confirm the first physician's diagnosis and treatment plan;

- confirm the first physician's diagnosis but offer one or more different treatment options or recommend slight changes to the original treatment plan; or

- in rare situations, provide a different diagnosis.

What a Second Opinion Is *Not*

It's also helpful to understand what a second opinion is *not*.

A second opinion is *not* an expression of distrust in your oncologist's judgment or abilities. Patients can have complete trust in their oncologist and still desire more input before making a decision. Physicians understand that patients may want to learn all they can before making decisions about their treatment.

A second opinion is *not* looking for a new physician. Patients who seek a second opinion usually visit the second physician, learn all they can, and then continue with their original oncologist.

A second opinion is *not* searching for a more desirable diagnosis. There have been situations where a person has trouble accepting the initial diagnosis, so he or she gets a second opinion hoping that the second physician will pronounce him or her cancer-free. Then, if that doesn't work, the person might seek out a third opinion—and then a fourth, and so on. Searching for a physician who will give better news is not in a patient's best interest.

Reasons Some People Seek a Second Opinion

People may seek a second opinion because they want another physician's assessment and ideas. An oncologist told me, "Medical professionals don't all look at things the same way, so a fresh set of eyes and a unique perspective can be very helpful in deciding on a course of treatment."

A second opinion can also help a patient feel more confident. One man described his experience this way:

> "My treatment plan indicated that a course of radiation was the only treatment I needed after surgery, but after talking it over with my doctor, I went for a second opinion just to be sure. The second doctor gave me an examination, looked over my medical records, read the pathology reports, answered my questions, and addressed my concerns. Then, after thorough analysis, he concurred with the treatment plan. The consultation really set my mind at ease as I proceeded with the original plan."

Reasons Some People Don't Seek a Second Opinion

Not everyone decides to get a second opinion. Some people might not get one because their medical team has indicated that they need to begin treatment immediately. Other patients may have already determined that the recommended treatment is the right one for them.

Questions and Answers about Second Opinions

Here are some questions people may have about second opinions, along with answers to consider.

Q: *If I get different information from the second opinion, how will I decide between the recommendations?*

You don't have to decide on your own. Your original oncologist can work with you to help decide which direction would be better for you. In addition, family or other loved ones will often be willing to help you think it through.

Q: *If I seek a second opinion, will I offend my oncologist?*

Most oncologists will not be offended by your asking about a second opinion. One told me, "I've never had an issue with patients wanting to get a second opinion. Diagnosing and treating cancer is complex, so I welcome the perspective of another physician."

Another physician had this to say: "As a patient, you should never be hesitant or concerned about getting a second opinion. In no way is it a dishonor or an insult to your physician when you seek one."

Q: *If I get a second opinion, am I saying I have doubts about my oncologist?*

Not at all. This point cannot be overstated: Oncologists know that getting a second opinion is not a sign of doubt but rather a helpful opportunity to get another perspective. Two opinions from medical experts are better than one. A physician told me how he benefits when a patient gets a second opinion that differs from his own recommendation:

"When a patient brings back a different recommendation from a second physician, I ask myself, *Why did Dr. B come up with a different opinion? What might this colleague have seen that I didn't?* Perhaps there's some information, data, or scientific study the other doctor has read that I haven't. Maybe that doctor has had experiences that I haven't had. I add the new information to what I already know, and I reanalyze the original treatment plan to see how I might improve it based on the new information."

Q: *Isn't it better to start cancer treatment right away? Wouldn't getting a second opinion hurt me by delaying the treatment I need?*

Not every cancer needs to be treated immediately; in fact, most patients have time to get a second opinion. If you need to start treatment right away, your oncologist will let you know.

Finding the Right Physician for a Second Opinion

Here are some thoughts about how to find a physician to provide you with a second opinion.

Ask Your Oncologist

Your first step is to talk with your oncologist and get his or her thoughts. One oncologist said, "The only caution I give my patients about second opinions is to get one from a reputable source. I'll gladly talk to patients about getting a second opinion and help them determine what would work best for them."

Consult Other Sources of Information

You might supplement what you learn from your oncologist with information from other sources about where to seek a second opinion. Here are some possibilities:

- Ask other medical professionals you're working with about physicians or medical facilities they would recommend for your second opinion.

- Use the resources in chapter 14, "Where to Look for Information about Your Kind of Cancer," to find potential sources for a second opinion.

- Check with your network of friends and allies, especially those who may have dealt with the same kind of cancer, and then run their suggestions past your medical team. One person said, "A friend from work who'd been through lymphoma sat down with my husband and me and shared suggestions about what we could do. She also suggested a doctor we could see for a second opinion. My oncologist spoke highly of the doctor my friend had recommended, so that's who I chose to see."

Reasons to Look outside Your Oncologist's Practice for a Second Opinion

If you decide to seek a second opinion, it can be a good idea to find a physician outside your oncologist's practice. Here are a few reasons:

- Your oncologist may have consulted with others in his or her practice before deciding on your treatment plan, so he or she may have already factored in their opinions. One survivor said, "My oncologist said up front that he reviewed my treatment plan with the other doctors in his office to make sure he'd taken everything into account. He recommended a doctor outside the practice for a second opinion to make sure I was getting a fresh perspective."

- Although this isn't always the case, sometimes physicians in the same practice tend to take similar treatment approaches. It can be beneficial to get your second opinion from an oncologist who may take a somewhat different approach.

- You may want to get your second opinion from a specialist or comprehensive cancer center that focuses on your specific kind of cancer.

- You may have greater peace of mind if this second opinion, coming from an independent source, confirms your diagnosis and treatment plan.

Working with the Physician Providing a Second Opinion

Before you meet with a second physician, he or she will need to review your test results, any pathology reports, and any medical images, such as CT scans, MRIs, or PET scans. Ask your oncologist to send these items to the second physician. It can also help to gather as many of these items as you can and take them with you to your appointment (see chapter 16, "Keeping Track of Personal Medical Information"). If you end up bringing information that the second physician already has, that's okay.

It's a good idea to call the second physician's office before the appointment to make sure your medical records have arrived. A nurse said, "Most of the time it isn't an issue, but just in case a glitch happens, a simple phone call to confirm that the physician got the records can save a lot of time, effort, and expense."

If you've compiled a summary or calendar with the details of your diagnosis and treatment, it can be helpful to share them with the second physician. These tools are described in chapter 16 and the appendix, "Chronological Diagnosis and Treatment Tracking Tools."

The physician may conduct an examination or order additional tests before giving a second opinion, or he or she may take a fresh look at the information that's already available and provide a second opinion based on that. In either situation, let the physician know of any changes you've experienced since the first opinion; the physician will want to take these into account in determining his or her own opinion.

When you meet the second physician, prepare thoroughly for the appointment so you can make the most of it. Bring a list of questions to ask, probably including many of the same questions you asked your oncologist (see chapter 13, "Medical Questions to Ask and When to Ask Them") as well as any additional questions you've thought of. If there are differences between the second opinion and the first, ask about the reasons for those differences.

It's a good idea to have someone come with you to provide a second set of ears during the conversation and perhaps ask additional questions. Even if you take careful notes, it's helpful for the other person to take notes as well. (See chapter 27, "Bring Someone with You to Appointments.")

Review the Second Opinion with Your Oncologist

Once you've obtained a second opinion, talk again with your original oncologist. Review what you've learned, weigh the options with him or her, and come to a decision.

It's your right to seek a second opinion or choose not to. If you decide to get a second or subsequent opinion, you can do so confidently, knowing that whatever the result—whether the physician confirms the initial plan or suggests new possibilities—you'll have additional information to use going forward.

20

Clinical Trials

"When I was diagnosed, my doctor suggested a clinical trial. I thought, 'Let's go for it. It will increase my chances—and it could help someone else later on.' Twenty years later, my son had the same cancer I had, and that experimental treatment had become the new standard. It saved both our lives."

Researchers are constantly working to advance cancer treatment. Clinical trials can be a way for you to get early access to these new treatments.

A physician told me, "I've been involved in conducting clinical trials for nearly 25 years. Back when I started, the treatments we were researching were cutting edge. After a while, many of them became the norm."

When you participate in a clinical trial, you work with physicians and other medical professionals who are committed to finding new cancer treatments. I spoke with a physician who has devoted his career to leading clinical trials. He had this to say about clinical trials and researchers:

> "Those of us who are designing and testing these treatments honestly and truly want to keep making cancer treatment better. There's a tremendous desire to help people. It's exciting to see all these treatments in development, knowing that some of them are going to make a difference with overall survival. We're all really passionate about finding new ways to fight cancer."

What Are Clinical Trials?

Clinical trials are research studies conducted by medical professionals to learn how to improve medical care for particular conditions. Most cancer-related clinical trials concentrate on treatments, measuring their safety and effectiveness. Others focus on prevention or detection. This chapter is about clinical trials that concentrate on cancer *treatment*.

Phases of Clinical Trials

Clinical trials typically move through three or four phases for a particular treatment being tested. Here are the main questions each phase seeks to answer.

Phase I Clinical Trials: Is the Treatment Safe?

Phase I clinical trials focus on finding out whether a new treatment is safe after it has shown promise in initial research.

> The main reason for doing phase I studies is to find the highest dose of the new treatment that can be given safely without serious side effects. . . . These studies also help to decide on the best way to give the new treatment. . . .
>
> Safety is the main concern at this point. Doctors keep a close eye on the people [involved in the clinical trial] and watch for any serious side effects.[1]

Phase II Clinical Trials: Does the Treatment Work?

The goal of a phase II clinical trial is to determine whether a new treatment has an effect on a certain kind of cancer.

> The type of benefit or response the doctors look for [in phase II clinical trials] depends on the goal of the treatment. It may mean the cancer shrinks or disappears. Or it might mean there's an extended period of time where the cancer doesn't get any bigger, or there's a longer time before the cancer comes back. In some studies, the benefit may be an improved quality of life. . . .
>
> If enough patients benefit from the treatment, and the side effects aren't too bad, the treatment is allowed to go on to a phase III clinical trial.[2]

Phase III Clinical Trials: Is the Treatment Better than What's Already Available?

Phase III trials are much broader than phase II trials and involve further tests to evaluate a new treatment's effectiveness.

---

1 "Clinical Trials: What You Need to Know," American Cancer Society, http://www.cancer.org/acs/groups/cid/documents/webcontent/003006-pdf.pdf, p. 8.

2 American Cancer Society, p. 9.

Treatments that have been shown to work in phase II studies usually must succeed in one more phase of testing before they're approved for general use. Phase III clinical trials compare the safety and effectiveness of the new treatment against the current standard treatment.

Because doctors do not yet know which treatment is better, study participants are often picked at random . . . to get either the standard treatment or the new treatment.[3]

After successful phase III clinical trials, a new treatment can be submitted for approval from the Food and Drug Administration (FDA).

Phase IV Clinical Trials: What Else Do We Need to Know?

Once a treatment has earned FDA approval and is being used effectively to treat cancer, it sometimes enters phase IV trials for additional research.

Even after testing a new medicine on thousands of people, the full effects of the treatment may not be known. Some questions may still need to be answered. For example . . . Are there rare side effects that haven't been seen yet, or side effects that only show up after a person has taken the drug for a long time? These types of questions may take many more years to answer, and are often addressed in phase IV clinical trials.[4]

In some phase IV studies, researchers explore whether a treatment approved for one type of cancer can be used effectively with patients who have a different kind of cancer.

Myths and Misconceptions about Clinical Trials

To make the best decision about participating in clinical trials, it's important to have an accurate understanding of them. Here are some widespread myths and misconceptions, followed by the facts.

Myth: *Only patients who have no other treatment options participate in clinical trials.*

Fact: Cancer patients can participate in clinical trials at any time during their treatment, as long as they meet the specific requirements for the trial. Many join a clinical trial as part of their initial treatment.

---

3 American Cancer Society, pp. 9–10.

4 American Cancer Society, pp. 10–11.

Myth: *Clinical trials are just wild experimentation.*

Fact: Clinical trials are tightly controlled experiments that must meet specific criteria. Before a clinical trial starts, researchers conduct rigorous studies to decide whether the treatment is likely to be effective against cancer. Then researchers seek approval from an institutional review board—an independent committee that includes physicians not involved in the clinical trial, nurses, scientists, community advocates, bioethicists, social workers, attorneys, and others. The board makes sure that the clinical trial adheres to all federal regulations and policies that protect participants. Once the trial is underway, the board works with the research team and the sponsoring organization to carefully monitor the study and safeguard participants' well-being. Regional and national organizations, including the FDA and the National Institutes of Health, also oversee clinical trials.

Myth: *Patients entering clinical trials have no idea what they're getting into.*

Fact: Prior to participating in a clinical trial, a patient will meet with a member of the research team conducting or coordinating the clinical trial. That research team member will explain every aspect of the trial, including how the trial will be conducted, possible benefits, and possible risks. He or she will address any questions or concerns the patient may have.

The research team member will give the patient written material about the clinical trial, including an *informed consent form,* which the patient may take home and review with loved ones. This document provides a great deal of information in plain, clear language to ensure that the patient knows everything he or she needs to know about the clinical trial. The patient will usually meet once more with a research team member to address any other questions or concerns before signing the informed consent form.

A physician heavily involved in clinical trials told me, "The informed consent form is a clearly spelled-out agreement between the patient, the clinician, and the organization sponsoring the clinical trial. It's about building trust and making it very clear what we're trying to do."

Myth: *Patients lose all their rights when they sign up for a clinical trial.*

Fact: Participants' rights are protected by federal law. The institutional review board evaluates and monitors all clinical trials to verify that they are conducted ethically and to safeguard the rights of participants.

Myth: *Patients have to stay in the trial no matter what.*

Fact: Patients may withdraw their informed consent and leave a clinical trial whenever they wish and for any reason. They have complete and final say over their participation in a clinical trial.

Myth: *You're guaranteed to receive more effective treatment for your cancer if you participate in a clinical trial.*

Fact: The treatment being tested is not guaranteed to be more effective than the current standard treatment. No treatment, regardless of whether it's standard or still in research, can guarantee a successful outcome.

Myth: *Some patients receive only placebos and miss out on real treatment.*

Fact: According to the National Cancer Institute's online dictionary of cancer terms, a placebo is "An inactive substance or treatment that looks the same as, and is given the same way as, an active drug or treatment being tested. The effects of the active drug or treatment are compared to the effects of the placebo."[5] The use of placebos in cancer clinical trials is rare, and if a clinical trial does use a placebo, it is carefully controlled by federal law. A placebo can be used in only two situations:

1. **When the clinical trial is comparing the current standard treatment *by itself* to the current standard treatment *plus* an experimental treatment.** In these instances, *every* participant receives the standard treatment, so no one is ever without the established best treatment. On top of that, participants may receive either the experimental treatment or a placebo.

2. **When the standard recommendation for a particular type or stage of cancer is not to treat it.** In these instances, participants may receive either the treatment being tested in the clinical trial or a placebo (although placebos aren't always used in such studies). Those who receive the placebo won't be missing out on a recommended treatment because no treatment is recommended in their situation.

If a placebo is part of the clinical trial design, those running the trial will let all patients know up front about the possibility of receiving a placebo.

---

5 http://www.cancer.gov/dictionary, s.v. "placebo."

Advantages of Participating in a Clinical Trial

Participating in a clinical trial can have a number of advantages:

- A clinical trial offers hope for a treatment that might work better than the standard treatment. One researcher said, "It doesn't matter how good current treatments for cancer are—we're always looking for ways to make them even better."

- New treatments being tested may be designed to target cancer cells more precisely while affecting other cells less, potentially resulting in more effective treatments with fewer side effects.

- You may benefit from a new form of treatment long before it's available for general use.

- Some clinical trials test combinations of the best available treatment plus the new treatment, which could enhance the overall effectiveness.

- Your participation in a clinical trial may help other patients in the future.

- Investigating and participating in a clinical trial can be a way to take action when your life may feel out of control. As a physician said, "Psychologically, it helps you feel like you're on offense rather than defense. That can make a big difference."

Another physician told me:

"One benefit patients receive from participating in a clinical trial is that they're going to be working even more closely with their healthcare providers. I give excellent care to each patient, but those who participate in clinical trials receive additional attention from the clinical researchers over and above what I'm able to give them."

Possible Challenges of Participating in a Clinical Trial

There are also some potential challenges to taking part in a clinical trial:

- It may take time and effort to find a suitable clinical trial.

- Even when you find a clinical trial for your type and stage of cancer, it's not guaranteed that you'll be able to participate. First, the study must be open for enrollment, meaning that it's still adding participants. Second, to be accepted into a study, you must meet all the specific requirements for that study.

- You might need to travel to participate in a clinical trial.

- You might have some additional expenses to cover if you participate, such as housing if the trial site is out of town.

- New medications or procedures may have risks and side effects. Participants are informed about these ahead of time and then are carefully monitored.

- Applying for and participating in a clinical trial may require more work for you and your family, such as additional office visits or tests.

If you have questions or concerns about participating in a clinical trial, talk with your medical team.

Finding a Clinical Trial

With more and more treatment facilities getting involved in cancer research, it's becoming easier to find clinical trials nearby, even if you don't live near a major cancer center. According to the National Cancer Institute:

> Cancer clinical trials take place in cities and towns across the United States and throughout the world. They take place in doctors' offices, cancer centers, medical centers, community hospitals and clinics, and veterans' and military hospitals. A single trial may take place in one or two places, or at hundreds of different sites.[6]

An oncologist said, "People often think they need to go to a large cancer center for a clinical trial, but because of how easily information is exchanged today, you can often participate at smaller hospitals and clinics."

If you're considering participating in a clinical trial, start by asking your oncologist, "Are there any clinical trials available right now that I might participate in?" He or she may know about current trials related to your type of cancer or may even be involved in conducting one. Your oncologist can help you determine which clinical trials you may be eligible for and whether any of them would be good for you to consider. Your medical team may also be able to help you with the enrollment process.

You, a family member, or a friend can also search the internet for information on clinical trials. Two places to look are the websites for the National Cancer Institute (NCI), cancer.gov, and the American Cancer

---

6 "Where Trials Take Place," National Cancer Institute,
   http://www.cancer.gov/about-cancer/treatment/clinical-trials/what-are-trials/where.

Society (ACS), cancer.org. Each website offers a user-friendly process for determining which clinical trials you might be eligible for and how to obtain more information about them. Both organizations also provide toll-free phone support for people exploring clinical trials (the NCI at 800-422-6237, the ACS at 800-227-2345).

Another valuable website is clinicaltrials.gov, operated by the National Institutes of Health. This site features an extensive database of clinical trials being conducted across the U.S. and around the world. You might use it to see what clinical trials are available for your kind of cancer and then discuss what you find with your medical team.

Once you've gathered information about possible clinical trials, share summaries of that information with your oncologist. The oncologist can help you look into and decide about the clinical trials you've identified, and he or she will be the one who connects you with a clinical trial if you choose to get involved.

Questions to Ask about a Clinical Trial

Here are some questions to ask about any clinical trial. You might come up with more.

1. **What is the purpose of the study?**

2. **Why do the researchers think the new treatment will be effective?**

3. **What are the eligibility requirements?**

4. **What does participating in the study require me to do? What expectations are there of me besides receiving the treatment?**

5. **Where will the clinical trial take place?**

6. **Will I need to be hospitalized? If so, how often and for how long?**

7. **Have there been prior clinical trials of this new treatment?**

8. **Will receiving this treatment affect my ability to receive other treatments?**

9. How long will it take to get started?

10. How long will the clinical trial last?

11. What short-term benefits should I look for? What long-term benefits?

12. What side effects can I expect? How will they be monitored and managed?

13. What costs might be involved?

14. What is the quality of my life likely to be during the clinical trial?

15. What risks does this treatment have?

16. How will I know whether the study treatment is working?

17. Who will be my main point of contact during the trial? How can I get in touch with that person?

You can find additional lists of questions to ask about clinical trials by using the search feature on the websites for the National Cancer Institute (cancer.gov) and the American Cancer Society (cancer.org).

Deciding Whether to Get Involved in a Clinical Trial

After learning more and weighing the pros and cons, some people decide to join a clinical trial and others don't.

One cancer survivor told me, "I decided to be part of a clinical trial because the treatment was showing a lot of promise. It gave me another way to fight back. Plus, it might help other people in the future."

Another said, "I chose not to participate in a clinical trial. My oncologist said that in my specific situation, the standard treatment on its own would be the best option."

Joining or not joining a clinical trial is a personal decision for each patient. Look at the clinical trials that are available, learn what you can, consult with your medical team, discuss your options with your loved ones, and make the best decision for your situation.

21

Pain Management

*You should never accept pain as a normal part
of having cancer. All pain can be treated, and
most pain can be controlled or relieved.*
–American Cancer Society[1]

Ongoing pain is not an inevitable part of cancer. Your medical team will
work with you and do everything possible to manage any pain you
might experience.

It's essential to deal with pain promptly and effectively. Unmanaged pain
can add to suffering and interfere with your healing. A nurse said, "When
you're in pain, it's difficult, if not impossible, to concentrate on anything else.
It's only when your pain is well managed that you'll be able to fully focus on
dealing with cancer."

Pain management is definitely not a one-size-fits-all treatment. It needs
to be customized for each patient. You are the key to helping your medical
team effectively manage your pain. That means it's important to understand
your pain and the management options available to you.

Types of Pain

Cancer-related pain usually falls into one of three categories.

Acute pain comes on quickly and lasts a relatively short time.

Persistent or chronic pain is constant or ongoing—either it doesn't go away
or it comes back frequently. Sometimes it's called background pain.

Breakthrough pain is a sharp, sudden spike of pain that, unlike acute
pain, occurs when a person is already taking medicine or using other means

---

1 "Guide to Controlling Cancer Pain," American Cancer Society,
   http://www.cancer.org/acs/groups/content/@editorial/documents/document/acspc-046379.pdf, p. 2.

to manage pain. Breakthrough pain might be brought on by a particular incident or activity, might flare up when the current dose of pain medication is wearing off, or may occur unpredictably for no identifiable reason. If it happens, it may be infrequent—perhaps once a week—or as frequent as several times a day.

Your medical team can help you manage any of these types of pain.

Causes of Pain

Pain may be caused by the cancer itself—for example, by a tumor pressing on a nerve or an organ. Pain also may come as a side effect of treatment or an aftereffect of surgery, a medical test, or a procedure. Some pain may be unrelated to the cancer, but it still should be discussed with your medical team and treated.

Methods of Pain Management

Methods for managing pain are constantly improving. Here are some of the main types available. Depending on your specific needs, you might use more than one of these methods.

Medications. Most people think first of opiate-derived drugs such as morphine and oxycodone for pain management, but these opioids aren't the only medications prescribed for pain. More familiar pain medications include acetaminophen and nonsteroidal anti-inflammatory drugs (NSAIDs) such as aspirin and ibuprofen; be sure to check with your medical team before using over-the-counter medicines like these. Other kinds of medications that are sometimes prescribed to help manage pain include steroids, antihistamines, antidepressants, muscle relaxants, and stimulants. They can come in many forms, including tablets, liquids, patches, sprays, patient-controlled pumps, and oral medications that dissolve under the tongue.

Nerve block. This is a procedure where medication is injected into or around a nerve or the spine in order to block pain.

Surgical intervention. Surgery to remove or reduce a tumor can be effective for managing pain.

Shrinking a tumor. Sometimes radiation or chemotherapy can help control pain by shrinking a tumor so that it doesn't press on organs or nerves.

For more about these and other methods of pain management, you can get a free booklet from the National Cancer Institute at cancer.gov or by calling 800-422-6237.

Speak Up about Your Pain

Medical professionals consider pain to be the fifth vital sign, after temperature, pulse, respiration, and blood pressure—it's an important indicator of what's going on in your body. Unlike those other vital signs, however, pain isn't something your medical team can measure. They need you to tell them about it. You are the authority on your pain. You are the only one who can say exactly where it hurts, when, and how much—so the key to getting help is to speak up.

Despite this, medical professionals have told me again and again that cancer patients often significantly *underreport* their pain. Across the board, medical professionals want patients to be straightforward and not hold back in describing their pain.

Reasons People May Be Reluctant to Talk about Their Pain

Sometimes people keep their pain to themselves instead of telling their medical team about it. Here are some common reasons.

"I don't want to seem like a complainer." Your medical team won't think that you're complaining when you report pain. One nurse said, "It's so important for patients to tell their medical team about their pain. We can't always tell when someone is in pain just by looking at the person. And we can't help with the pain unless we know about it." An oncologist agreed, saying, "People shouldn't be afraid to tell us when they're in pain or if our efforts to keep their pain under control aren't working. The most rewarding part of our job is being able to help people, and we can do that most effectively when they let us know that they're hurting."

"I don't want to appear weak." Telling your medical team about your pain is not a sign of weakness. On the contrary, letting your medical team know about your pain shows personal strength and demonstrates trust that your medical team will listen and provide the help you need.

"Others tolerate pain, so I should too." It doesn't do any good to compare your pain tolerance with that of others. Enduring pain is not a contest, and there are no prizes for the person who toughs it out the longest. Everyone has personal tolerance levels for different kinds of pain. Know your own tolerance levels so you can ask for help early—before the pain increases so much that it becomes difficult to manage.

"I don't want to worry my loved ones or make them uncomfortable by admitting that I'm in pain." Your loved ones want to see you get the best care possible, including treatment for any pain you have. When you get the help you need to manage your pain, you'll do a lot more to ease their worries than if you try to hide or downplay what you're going through. Plus, when you're honest and open with your loved ones about your pain, they can help you keep track of it or communicate about it with your medical team.

"My pain has changed, and I'm worried about what this change might mean." If a person's pain changes, perhaps by becoming more intense or moving to a different spot, fear of what the change means may make that person reluctant to bring it up. But the only effective way to deal with this fear is to address the uncertainty and tell your medical team about the changes you notice. When you let the team know about changes to your pain, you help them get a better picture of what you're experiencing, which enables them to manage your pain most effectively.

"This pain probably isn't related to the cancer treatment, so I shouldn't bother my oncologist about it." Even if you don't think a pain is related to cancer, mention it to your medical team anyway. If it turns out to be non-cancer pain, managing it still offers relief and strengthens your ability to deal with cancer. Your medical team may be able to do something about it, or they may refer you to another physician to treat it.

"I don't want to get addicted to pain medication." Your medical team can help you use pain medications properly to minimize the risk of addiction. The American Cancer Society states:

> Addiction is a common fear of people taking pain medicine. Such fear may keep you from taking the medicine. Or it may cause family members to encourage you to hold off as long as you can between doses.

> Addiction is defined as uncontrollable drug craving, seeking, and continued use. When opioids (also known as narcotics)—the strongest pain relievers available—are taken for pain, they rarely cause addiction as defined here. When you're ready to stop taking opioids, the doctor will lower the amount of medicine you're taking over a few days or weeks. By the time you stop using it completely, your body has had time to

adjust. Talk to your cancer care team about how to take pain medicines safely and about any concerns you have about addiction.[2]

"I don't want to deal with the side effects of pain medication." Side effects of pain medicine, just like side effects of cancer treatment, can be managed if you work with your medical team to address them. Chapter 22, "Side Effects," says more about this.

"If I take pain medication now, it might become ineffective later." While the body can build a tolerance to some medications, your medical team can use a variety of approaches, including changing, alternating, or combining medications, as well as adjusting dosages, to treat pain effectively over the long term if needed.

"I don't want to feel drowsy or sleep all the time." Pain medications can cause drowsiness for some people. If they make you drowsy, the effect will often subside as your body adjusts to the medication. Furthermore, when you let your medical team know what's happening, they can help manage the effect, possibly by changing the dosage or type of medication.

Discuss any questions or concerns you have about pain management with your medical team. Don't let anything keep you from talking about your pain.

What Can Happen When People Don't Talk about Their Pain

When people don't speak up about their pain, they're less likely to get help managing it. Here are some of the consequences of unmanaged pain.

Less enjoyment of life. People in pain tend to pull back from activities they would otherwise enjoy.

Diminished mental abilities. Pain might interfere with a person's ability to think clearly, focus on a task, and remember accurately.

Decreased hope. Unmanaged pain can cause people to become discouraged and pessimistic.

Difficult emotions. Constant pain can generate strong, difficult emotions such as intense anger, fear, anxiety, or sadness.

---

2 "Guide to Controlling Cancer Pain," American Cancer Society, http://www.cancer.org/acs/groups/content/@editorial/documents/document/acspc-046379.pdf, pp. 6–7.

Immobility. Those in pain may be less likely to get up and move around. Persistent immobility can lead to diminished strength, decreased blood flow, constipation, and other health problems.

Delays in addressing complications. Pain can indicate a complication, such as an infection. The longer a person waits to tell his or her medical team about the pain, the more serious that complication might become.

Reduced interaction with family and friends. When a person is in pain, he or she may not feel like talking to anyone and can become isolated. When someone does talk with him or her, the person in pain may find it hard to concentrate on the conversation and may not get much enjoyment out of it.

Increased stress on relationships. If someone has uncontrolled pain, his or her loved ones are often concerned and anxious. They want to help but feel powerless to do so. The resulting frustration, combined with the ongoing pain, can cause stress and tension to increase, which can strain relationships.

Here's how one nurse summed up the problems with not talking about pain:

> "When a patient tries to endure the pain, there's a snowball effect—pain builds up, causing other issues such as restlessness, sleeplessness, fatigue, immobility, a loss of appetite, and isolation. Unreported pain can hurt the patient's overall situation."

Work with Your Medical Team to Manage the Pain

Managing pain requires a team effort, and you are the most important member of the team. Here's how you and your loved ones can work with your medical team regarding your pain and its treatment.

Don't Wait to Deal with Your Pain

Contact your medical team as soon as pain occurs or if it appears to be getting worse despite pain management efforts. Don't hesitate or wait for your next appointment to deal with your pain. An oncology nurse said, "If a new pain develops, call right away. We can help you if you'll let us know what's going on."

Describe Your Pain

When you feel pain, it's important to let your medical team know exactly what you're experiencing. The more accurately you can describe your pain, and the more detail you can provide, the better your medical team can help you manage it.

Keep a Pain Journal

It can be helpful to keep a journal to track your pain. In that journal, you might include:

- Where you feel the pain, where it seems to be coming from, and whether it moves over time.
- Whether it's acute, persistent, or breakthrough pain, as described on page 103.
- When the pain begins.
- What you were doing before or when the pain started.
- What the pain feels like—use descriptive words like *sharp, radiating, pounding, deep, dull, throbbing,* or *stabbing.*
- How intense the pain is, using a scale from 0 to 10—where 0 is no pain and 10 is the worst pain. Be candid about the intensity of the pain; if it's an 8, 9, or 10, don't hesitate to say that. Include lower-intensity pains too, because they may be part of a pattern—and it's easier to manage pain when you can catch it early. Also, try to rate pain levels consistently so your medical team will know how your pain one day compares to your pain another day.

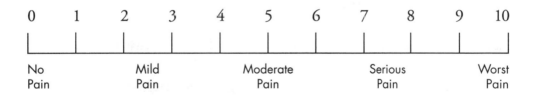

- When the pain peaks.
- When the pain lessens or ends.
- What makes the pain worse or better.
- Any medications or other pain management techniques (such as ice, heat, or massage) you use, when you use them, what effect they have on the pain, and how long the effect lasts.

A family member or caregiver can help you track your pain and keep your pain journal up to date.

There are also tools available online and for mobile devices to help you keep track of your pain and then generate a report to take to your next appointment. A web search using the keywords *pain tracking tool* can show you what's available. Tools like these can make it easier to track your pain and tell your medical team about it.

Take your pain journal to your appointments to show your medical team what your pain is like now and how it's changed over time.

Questions to Ask about Your Pain Medications

If a pain medication is prescribed, make sure you get answers to questions such as the following:

1. **How much should I take, when, and how?**

2. **How long does it take for the medicine to start working? How long should each dose last?**

3. **What should I do if the pain comes back before it's time for the next dose?**

4. **What should I do if I forget to take my medications or if I get off schedule?**

5. **Are there any medications or supplements I should avoid while I'm taking this medicine?**

6. **Are there any foods I need to avoid while taking this medicine?**

7. **Is it safe to drink alcohol while using this medicine?**

8. **Is it safe to drive while using this medicine?**

9. **Are there any other safety issues to keep in mind while using this medicine?**

10. **What are the side effects of this medicine, and how can I prevent or deal with them?**

11. **If I have questions, whom should I call?**

12. **What symptoms, problems, or reactions should I call about right away?**

In addition to your medical team, your pharmacist can be an excellent source of information for these questions.

Stick to the Pain Management Plan

An essential part of keeping pain under control is to follow the pain management plan you've established with your medical team.

If you have a specific schedule for taking a medication, follow it. Your pain management plan is designed to keep ahead of pain—to prevent it from becoming difficult to control. If you think you may not need the pain medication any longer, or if you think you need stronger or more frequent medication, talk about it with your medical team instead of making any changes on your own.

If your medical team has given you pain medication to take as needed, take it according to the directions. By taking the medication as directed, you can help keep the pain under control so it doesn't have a chance to get worse.

Don't wait until you're in a pain crisis before you address the pain. Here's what a nurse told me:

> "When a patient puts off dealing with pain and ends up in a pain crisis, the pain is much harder to manage. It's harder for the patient to think clearly, respond accurately to questions about the pain, and assess the impact of pain medications. Likewise, it's harder for the patient's family to contribute to a conversation about pain management when they're upset over their loved one's pain and they urgently want the pain relieved. It's also harder for the medical team to know which pain medications will work best for the patient because we haven't had the opportunity to try a variety of them when the pain was less severe."

Family members who help patients take their pain medications also need to support the pain management plan. One nurse put it this way:

> "Family members are susceptible to the same worries and concerns as patients when it comes to pain medications. But it's important that they not waver or take it upon themselves to make medication decisions that may not be in the patient's best interest. So if family members have any questions or uncertainties, they need to talk to the

medical team so we can address those issues, help them understand the plan, change the plan as necessary, and encourage them to stay committed to it."

You are the expert on any pain you experience, and you have the right to have your pain acknowledged and treated. Through clear, honest communication, you and your medical team can become effective partners against pain.

22

Side Effects

*"My nurses and doctors encouraged me to tell
them about all my side effects. So every time
a problem occurred, I brought it up with them
and got help dealing with it. I figured,
'Why suffer if I don't have to?'"*

Cancer treatment can result in side effects—unintended consequences
that are not caused by the cancer itself but by the medications and
procedures used to treat the disease. These side effects can be uncomfortable
or even distressing at times.

However, when you work with your medical team, they'll be able to help
you manage and reduce most side effects—and even minimize or prevent
some of them before they happen. One nurse said, "You don't have to tolerate
side effects or stop the treatment that's causing them. There are ways around
many side effects. Let us know if you're experiencing something, and we'll
do whatever we can to help."

This chapter provides an overview of side effects, suggestions for learning more about them, and information about the role you can play in
managing them.

Kinds of Side Effects

The following is an alphabetical listing of some of the possible side effects
of cancer treatments. You can find out from your medical team what side
effects might be possible for a specific treatment. Your team can give you
suggestions about how to manage the side effects.

The type of side effects you may experience will be unique to you and
your situation; each person might have some side effects and not have others.
In addition, many side effects are temporary and will go away once your
treatment is complete.

Allergic Reactions

An infrequent side effect is an allergic reaction to a cancer treatment. Such reactions can be serious and can limit the types of treatment a person may safely receive. It's important to let your medical team know about your allergies and find out what symptoms of an allergic reaction to watch for.

Cognitive Issues

Sometimes cancer treatments can cause temporary issues with memory, concentration, language, or thinking clearly. You may be able to cope with these side effects by using techniques to help with memory (for example, writing down or recording things you want to remember), getting help from friends and family, and getting regular exercise for your body and mind. It can also be good to take things more slowly and be cautious when doing certain activities. Above all, go easy on yourself.

Cold or Heat

Some treatments can cause patients to feel extremely cold or hot. One person said, "After chemo, it could go either way—sometimes I had chills, other times I was sweating."

Dehydration

During treatment, dehydration can occur because of multiple factors, including loss of appetite, nausea, diarrhea, and the inability to keep fluids down. This side effect can become serious if untreated, so it's important to talk about it with your medical team. It may be possible to address this side effect through nutritional changes or by getting fluids intravenously.

Diarrhea or Constipation

Digestive side effects, including diarrhea and constipation, are possible with some cancer treatments. If you experience digestive problems, talk with your medical team about steps you can take to lessen the side effect, including adjusting your diet. Also, consult with the team before taking any over-the-counter medicines such as laxatives; sometimes such medications can cause additional problems.

Emotional Effects

Side effects can be emotional as well as physical. During treatment, people may experience different kinds of emotional distress, including anxiety, mood swings, and depression. Emotional effects can come as a direct result of the treatment or in response to a side effect, such as when patients struggle with self-image due to changes in their appearance. Part 2 of this book includes more details about the emotional effects of cancer.

Pay attention to your emotional state and note any significant changes—or ask a loved one to do this—so you can get help from your medical team before the emotional effects become severe.

Fatigue

Cancer patients may experience fatigue. It's not uncommon for a person to lack energy even after getting plenty of sleep, especially in the days following a treatment. Fatigue may occur right away or peak several days later.

Often fatigue can be addressed through lifestyle changes, such as being consistent with your rest periods, maintaining a balanced diet, or engaging in light exercise on a regular basis. After you finish treatment, it's likely that your energy will gradually return.

Hair Loss

Chemotherapy often results in alopecia, or hair loss, but not always. The timing and extent of hair loss varies from person to person. It may occur gradually or rapidly and can range from thinning hair to losing all the hair on one's body.

Radiation therapy can also cause hair loss. Typically, the loss is localized to the area of the body receiving radiation treatment.

After treatment has ended, hair will generally start growing back, possibly with a new texture or color. Often, the difference is only temporary.

It's possible to prepare for hair loss and control how it affects you. See the section called "Be Prepared" on page 118 of this chapter.

Infection

Because cancer treatments such as chemotherapy and radiation can weaken the immune system, a patient may be more susceptible to infection. The best defense against infection is practicing careful hygiene, including regular hand-washing and showering, and maintaining a healthy diet. Depending on your situation, you may be advised to limit your exposure to crowds or other environments where people may be ill. If you notice any signs of infection (such as fever, coughing, sore throat, redness, swelling, or pain), report them to your medical team immediately.

Nausea and Vomiting

Advances in treatment and anti-nausea medications have made nausea and vomiting less common and less severe, but it remains a possibility with chemo-therapy and some radiation treatments. You may receive a prescription for an anti-nausea medication as well as suggestions for adjusting your diet or eating patterns to reduce the occurrence of these symptoms.

Oral Complications

Sometimes treatment causes people to experience various oral complications, such as dry mouth, increased sensitivity to cold foods and beverages, mouth sores, an unpleasant taste in their mouth, or other dental problems. These complications can also affect a person's appetite and comfort. You can minimize many of these issues by practicing good oral hygiene and avoiding specific foods as suggested by your medical team; other problems may be treated through medications.

If at all possible, before starting treatment, get a dental checkup so you can let your dentist know about the treatment and take care of any dental issues that could become sources of infection. It's also good to get any necessary dental work done before treatment begins. If dental needs arise during treatment, consult with both your medical team and your dentist about how best to deal with them.

Pain

Some cancer treatments cause pain, but it can be managed to a large degree. This subject is covered in chapter 21, "Pain Management."

Peripheral Neuropathy

Peripheral neuropathy is caused by damage to nerves outside the brain and spinal cord. Symptoms can include pain, tingling, burning, cold, or numbness in the feet or hands. As a result, some people may have difficulty walking or performing fine motor functions like buttoning a shirt. These symptoms can be temporary or ongoing. Talk with your medical team about possible treatments.

Skin and Nail Issues

Some patients may experience rashes, itching, swelling, dryness, or other skin problems. Fingernails and toenails can become thin, brittle, or discolored.

Where to Learn More about Possible Side Effects

As you learn about your kind of cancer and possible treatments using the approaches described in chapter 14, "Where to Look for Information about Your Kind of Cancer," you'll probably come across information about side effects. The side effects you're most likely to encounter will depend in part on your course of treatment, so look for information about side effects specific to your treatment plan.

The following are some effective sources for learning more about side effects.

Your Medical Team

The first step is always to ask your oncologist about the side effects you might experience. See chapter 13, "Medical Questions to Ask and When to Ask Them," for a list of questions to ask about possible side effects.

An oncology nurse, nurse practitioner, or physician's assistant on your team is also a good person to ask. Because these professionals work so closely with patients, they're especially familiar with side effects, the kinds of questions people have about them, and ways to deal with them. Pharmacists can be another good source of information on side effects of medications, as well as options for handling those side effects.

Others Who Have Experience with Your Treatment

You might get suggestions about managing side effects by asking people who have experience with the treatment you're receiving. However, everyone responds to treatments differently, and patients' treatment plans may be highly individualized, so another person's experiences with side effects won't necessarily match up with yours.

It's important to check with your medical team before you try any remedies, including over-the-counter medications or supplements.

Cancer Associations

The American Cancer Society (cancer.org) and the National Cancer Institute (cancer.gov) have literature about side effects. A way to get general information is to just enter the words *side effects* into the search bar on either website. You might also conduct a narrower search by entering the words *side effects* plus a particular side effect or the name of a medication or other treatment that you are receiving.

Information from Pharmaceutical Companies

A potentially helpful place to learn about possible side effects of a medication is directly from the company that developed it. You can usually get a pamphlet on the medication from your oncologist or pharmacist, or you can check the pharmaceutical company's website to find information about the medication.

You may also obtain helpful information from the inserts that come in medication packages. Be aware, however, that these inserts are typically written in technical language and list every known side effect, including many that are rare. Check with your medical team or your pharmacist if you're uncertain or concerned about anything.

Managing Your Side Effects

Knowing about possible side effects gives you and your medical team the opportunity to manage them as effectively as possible.

Be Prepared

If you're aware of what side effects are possible for your specific treatments, you can plan ahead to reduce their impact before they happen. For instance:

- If you plan on wearing a wig, many people recommend getting one before you begin chemotherapy so you can match it to your current hair and have it ready to go. You can also take the opportunity to change your look. I heard from one woman who had auburn hair but decided to wear a blonde wig during treatment, and she enjoyed the change.

- If fatigue is a likely side effect, it may help to arrange ahead of time for people to drive you to and from treatment appointments.

- If your treatment may limit your ability to eat or digest certain foods, you can begin planning meals that you'll most likely be able to handle.

One person said, "Knowing about the possible side effects made them seem scary at first. But it helped to be prepared for at least some of them—wig obtained, food on hand to eat, and helpers ready."

You can't plan for every possible side effect, but if you prepare for what is more likely to happen, you'll also be in a better position to handle other side effects that may occur.

Keep a Log

You may find it valuable to keep a log of the side effects you experience so you can provide your medical team with precise information. When a side effect occurs, write down the date, time, type of side effect, and any key details, including duration and severity. Use a consistent scale to describe the severity, possibly from 1 to 10, with 1 being extremely mild and 10 being extremely intense. Also record anything done to alleviate the side effect and what the result was.

The American Cancer Society website, cancer.org, has side effects worksheets that you can download, print, and use to track your side effects. You may also want to search online for tools to record side effects and organize information on your computer or mobile device.

Keep Your Medical Team Informed

Your medical team can help you manage the side effects you may encounter. They can also help you prepare for side effects and may be able to take steps to limit them before symptoms even appear.

If you're experiencing what may be a side effect, bring it up right away with your medical team. Immediate relief may be available. Don't try to handle it on your own, and don't wait to see whether it gets better or worse. Give your medical team the details of what you're experiencing. If you've been keeping a log, you can use it to show them a complete picture of your side effects. The more they know, the more they can help you.

Sometimes people think, *Of course I feel bad, I'm going through cancer treatment,* so they decide not to bother their medical team about the side effects they're experiencing. Here are four good reasons not to tough it out but instead to communicate with your medical team about any side effects you encounter:

1. Ignoring a side effect won't make it go away.

2. A side effect may be treatable. Dealing with it is an opportunity to make your life a little easier and relieve you from needless suffering.

3. Occasionally a side effect could be an indication of a more serious problem, such as an infection, a drug interaction, or an allergic reaction—all of which require immediate attention.

4. Side effects can make it more difficult to keep to your treatment plan, which may affect your treatment results.

Side effects may be a part of treatment—but they're a part you can have some control over. The more you learn and the more closely you work with your medical team, the better you can manage side effects. As one person told me, "Know as much as possible so you'll be prepared. It's not as scary when you know what may be coming."

23

Palliative Care

*"Palliative care was a godsend. It helped me **feel** better, which helped me fight harder to **get** better."*

As you are dealing with cancer, palliative care can provide help and support to make you more comfortable, more focused, and more effective. The National Cancer Institute defines palliative care this way:

> Palliative care is care given to improve the quality of life of patients who have a serious or life-threatening disease, such as cancer. The goal of palliative care is to prevent or treat, as early as possible, the symptoms and side effects of the disease and its treatment, in addition to the related psychological, social, and spiritual problems. . . . Palliative care is also called *comfort care, supportive care,* and *symptom management.*[1]

Questions and Answers about Palliative Care

The following questions and answers offer more details about what palliative care is and does.

Q: *Is palliative care the same thing as hospice care?*

Palliative care and hospice care are related, but there are differences between the two.

Hospice care is typically for patients with a life-limiting illness when the emphasis shifts from curing or controlling the disease to giving support and comfort to patients and their loved ones. It incorporates the principles and many of the practices of palliative care to help them live each day as fully as possible.

---

1 "Palliative Care in Cancer," National Cancer Institute, http://www.cancer.gov/cancertopics/factsheet/support/palliative-care.

Palliative care, as described by the National Cancer Institute, can help any cancer patient, no matter what the goal is for treatment. Whether patients are pursuing treatment to cure their cancer or to keep it at bay for a period of time, they can receive palliative care to help manage symptoms and side effects and to make their lives as comfortable as possible.

Q: *When can a patient receive palliative care?*

Any patient with cancer or another serious disease may receive palliative care at any time following the diagnosis. Palliative care can be offered along with treatment aimed at curing or controlling a person's cancer.

Q: *What kinds of support does palliative care provide for cancer patients?*

Palliative care involves working with the patient and his or her family to address their overall needs and desires. To that end, it can encompass many types of care and support, including:

- medication and other treatments and therapies to relieve pain, symptoms, and side effects such as loss of appetite, nausea, constipation, fatigue, difficulty sleeping, or shortness of breath

- attention to emotional, spiritual, and social needs, possibly involving professional counseling, talking with a chaplain about spiritual challenges, help with family communication, and other kinds of support and guidance

- help with practical needs such as navigating insurance and financial issues and connecting with agencies that provide assistance

The specific types of care will vary from person to person, since palliative care is tailored to the unique needs of the person receiving it.

Q: *Is palliative care just for patients?*

No—the patient's loved ones can also receive palliative care. They may benefit from emotional and spiritual support, guidance on ways to cope with and manage caregiver stress, respite services that give some time off to those providing care, and practical assistance with administrative, legal, and financial issues. One person said, "The people on Mom's palliative care team are just as supportive for the rest of the family as they are for her. They're great, caring listeners, and they offer much-needed advice about how to support Mom while also taking care of ourselves."

Q: How do I get palliative care?

If you're considering palliative care, start by bringing up the topic with your oncologist. Ask about what elements of palliative care are appropriate for your situation and how you can access them. Once you connect with those involved in providing palliative care, you can learn more from them about what kinds of palliative care are available.

Q: Who provides palliative care?

Your oncologist will take an active role in pain relief and symptom management. He or she may also consult with or involve other medical professionals who focus on specific areas of palliative care, such as nurse practitioners, physical therapists, social workers, pharmacists, dietitians, chaplains, counselors, and others who can help meet the varied needs of the patient and family members.

Q: What are the benefits of palliative care?

Palliative care can provide patients and their loved ones with a number of benefits, including:

Greater comfort. The American Society of Clinical Oncology recommends palliative care as a way to make a patient's cancer treatment easier overall: "Patients who receive palliative care at the same time as cancer treatment often have less severe symptoms, better quality of life, and report that they are more satisfied with treatment."[2]

More strength and energy. A nurse said:

> "Fighting pain and other symptoms can leave a person drained. Palliative care frees up the patient's energy by relieving pain and other symptoms. I had one patient who was in severe pain and had become lethargic and withdrawn. After receiving additional medication and treatment through palliative care to address the pain, his energy returned, and he was able to participate more fully in his treatment. The difference was like night and day."

Emotional release and relief. Social workers, counselors, chaplains, and other caring professionals provide palliative care by helping patients and

---

2 "ASCO Recommends Palliative Care as a Part of Cancer Treatment," American Society of Clinical Oncology, http://www.cancer.net/publications-and-resources/asco-care-and-treatment-recommendations-patients/asco-recommends-palliative-care-part-cancer-treatment.

family members with the emotional challenges that come with cancer. A hospital director said, "Even when patients are doing well physically, their level of stress or anxiety can be through the roof. Palliative care professionals specialize in providing support for those emotional difficulties."

Spiritual support. Chaplains can also help patients and family members with spiritual challenges, listening compassionately and providing a safe place to share.

A sense of control. A cancer patient told me, "The counseling and spiritual support I received as part of palliative care helped me to take control over some aspects of my life and cancer journey. I felt like a whole person, not just a disease or room number."

Less worry for family members. As palliative care provides relief and support for the patient, it can reduce family members' worries. A parent of a cancer patient said, "All of us benefited from the palliative care my daughter received. Just seeing how it helped her as she went through treatment eased a lot of our stress and gave us a sense of relief."

Q: *Where can I learn more about palliative care?*

A good place to find information is getpalliativecare.org, which includes a number of resources for learning more.

Palliative Care Helps Patients and Their Families

A nurse told me, "Palliative care can help patients and their families in so many ways—pain management, side-effect reduction, emotional care, family support. For many people, it gives the best chance for the best possible outcome."

Palliative care can be a great addition to your overall strategy. As one cancer survivor put it, "Just because you have cancer doesn't mean you have to feel like crap if there are ways not to."

Part 5

Alternative or Complementary Therapies

24

Defining and Describing Alternative and Complementary Therapies

"Complementary" and "alternative" are terms used to describe many kinds of products, practices, and systems that are not part of mainstream medicine.
–American Cancer Society[1]

In addition to conventional medical treatments, you may hear about nonstandard treatments referred to as *alternative* or *complementary* medicine.

Alternative medicine includes nonstandard practices that are used *instead of* conventional means of treatment. It involves replacing standard cancer treatment with other approaches.

Complementary medicine can include the same nonstandard practices as alternative medicine, but they're used *in addition to* standard cancer treatment. The person continues to receive standard cancer treatment but also adds one or more nonconventional approaches.

---

1 "Complementary and Alternative Methods and Cancer," American Cancer Society, http://www.cancer.org/acs/groups/cid/documents/webcontent/acspc-041660-pdf.pdf, p. 1.

Nonstandard practices—whether used to replace standard treatment or in addition to it—can generally be divided into five categories. The therapies mentioned in this chapter are listed only as examples; be sure to consult with your oncologist before pursuing any kind of treatment or therapy.

1. Diet

This includes eating or drinking certain things and avoiding others. Some examples are:

* Avoiding processed foods, red meat, or sugar
* Fish oil
* Green tea
* Herbal supplements
* Juices
* Prebiotics
* Probiotics
* Raw vegetables
* Vitamin and mineral supplements
* Whole grains

2. Exercise

This category involves performing certain physical actions or movements. Examples include:

* Aerobics
* Dance
* Pilates
* Resistance, range-of-motion, and strength training
* Swimming or water aerobics
* Tai chi
* Walking
* Yoga

3. Physical Treatments

This category includes manipulation or other body-based treatments, such as:

* Acupressure
* Acupuncture
* Heat and cold
* Massage

4. Mental or Emotional

These treatments focus on affecting the body through one's thoughts and feelings. Examples are:

* Art therapy
* Biofeedback
* Guided imagery
* Hypnosis
* Laughter therapy
* Meditation
* Music therapy
* Relaxation

5. Energy

These are based on the belief that controlling certain energy fields can affect the body. Examples include:

* Healing touch
* Magnet therapy
* Pulsed electromagnetic fields

The next two chapters offer some thoughts about nonstandard approaches.

25

Ask First

*"My friend was interested in some nonstandard
treatments, so she checked with her oncologist
before she did anything. She wanted to make sure
that it wouldn't have any negative effects
on her medical treatment."*

If you're considering any alternative or complementary treatment, ask your
oncologist about that treatment first.

Why Ask Your Oncologist First?

Some nonstandard treatments can have significant risks. Here are just a few
examples:

- Some herbal therapies can increase the effects of anticoagulants
  (sometimes referred to as blood thinners) and possibly cause internal
  bleeding.

- Vigorous or deep tissue massage can cause health risks for people with
  certain blood disorders.

- Taking large doses of certain vitamins can interfere with some types of
  chemotherapy.

Other nonstandard treatments may have serious risks as well. Your oncologist can let you know about such risks when you tell him or her about any
additional therapies you're considering.

An oncology nurse said, "Fighting cancer takes a delicate balance—
keeping in mind the cancer itself, the treatments, the side effects, the
treatments for the side effects—and if you change one thing, like adding a
nonstandard treatment, it can affect something else. That's why you always
need to check with your medical team before doing anything different."

When and How to Ask

Talk with your oncologist *before* you try any nonstandard treatment you may be considering. Bring along any information you have gathered about that treatment—because, as one oncology nurse mentioned, "There are so many nontraditional treatments out there, and more coming up every day, that your oncologist may not have heard about what you want to discuss." (See chapter 30, "Share Streamlined Information," for ideas about how best to put together information to share with your oncologist.)

One oncologist shared her view: "When it comes to any nonstandard treatment, the most important thing is making sure it doesn't have negative effects and the patient continues with the prescribed treatment that has been shown to be effective. That's why I urge patients to talk to me about it first."

26

Three Categories for Considering Suggestions

"They made a big show of concern—
'I'm worried about you, and I just wanted
to share some information I found.'
Then came the sales pitch."

People may approach you with suggestions for various nonstandard treatments—alternative or complementary. It can be tempting to try out the suggested treatments right away. As one survivor said, "When you're in the midst of a situation this frightening, any new possibility for getting better can be incredibly enticing. Plus, it's easy to feel guilty if you don't try something that someone has suggested—you can worry that you aren't doing everything possible to beat the cancer."

Consult with your medical team if you're considering any of these recommendations. In addition, it's a good idea to assess where the suggestion came from.

People who suggest nonstandard treatments generally fall into one of three categories. These categories can help indicate what the person's interests may be.

1. Someone Who *Has* Used the Treatment and Would Not Benefit Financially by Your Using It

A person in the first category recommends a treatment that:

    1. he or she is personally using or has used; and

    2. he or she wouldn't profit from if you used it.

I consider this to have the most merit of the three categories. The person genuinely believes that the treatment has helped, and he or she wants to pass those benefits along to others.

Of course, that doesn't guarantee that the treatment will be a good one for you. Even when people have good intentions, they may not always have a clear idea of how effective a treatment is or what would be best for you. As mentioned in chapter 25, "Ask First," always check with your oncologist if you're considering any nonstandard treatment.

2. Someone Who *Has Not* Used the Treatment and Would Not Benefit Financially by Your Using It

A person in the second category recommends a treatment that:

1. he or she hasn't used; and

2. he or she wouldn't profit from if you used it.

The person heard about the treatment somehow and decided to tell you about it.

Because the person has no experience using the treatment, the information is less reliable than it would be coming from a person in the first category. But because the person has no financial stake and no connection with the people selling the treatment, the potential conflict of interest is minimal.

3. Someone Who Would Benefit Financially by Your Using the Treatment

A person in the third category recommends a treatment that he or she would benefit financially from if you used it. The person might be a distributor or a sales representative for the treatment. He or she may or may not have used the treatment—the key factor is that the person would profit from your use of it and, therefore, has a significant conflict of interest. That factor doesn't necessarily disqualify what the person is suggesting; it simply means that you need to look very, very carefully at whose best interests he or she has in mind.

Respond Based on the Category

Whenever someone recommends a nonstandard treatment, ask yourself which of these three categories the person falls into. Doing so can help you decide how much consideration to give to the recommendation. Then, if you think it might be worth a closer look, discuss it with your medical team.

Some people, especially in the third category, might be tenacious about trying to get you to use a certain treatment. They may keep pressuring you and refuse to take no for an answer. If this happens, I encourage you to stand firm and say that you aren't interested—more than once if necessary. You can also ask a family member or friend to help you say no if you aren't comfortable with doing so yourself. (See chapter 60, "Say No," for suggestions about how to say no clearly and respectfully in a variety of situations.)

Considering which category the suggestion fits into can help you figure out how best to respond.

Part 6

Working with and Relating to Your Medical Team

27

Bring Someone with You to Appointments

"My friend was my second pair of ears and my second memory. After appointments, I was surprised at how much she'd heard and written down that I didn't remember."

I f possible, it's best to take a family member or friend with you to your appointments. That way you'll have two minds taking in what your physician tells you.

When you're dealing with cancer, it can sometimes be difficult to think clearly and remember everything your physician says or all the questions you need to ask. Having a family member or friend with you at your appointments can help you capture vital information and get the answers you need.

One person diagnosed with cancer told me, "During the first few meetings with my oncologist, I was still in shock and had trouble processing it all. I needed my friend with me to hear what was actually being said so I could ask him about it later."

A family member of another patient said, "Dad was nearly as overwhelmed by Mom's cancer as she was, so I went along with them to each doctor's appointment to write down instructions, help get their questions answered, and provide emotional support."

Many medical professionals have emphasized how important this is. An oncology nurse told me:

"I encourage all my patients to have someone with them at appointments. You need another set of ears, another set of eyes, another brain, because you may only catch half of what's said. It can be a friend, a spouse, or another family member—just have someone come to appointments with you."

Qualities of an Effective Person to Take with You to Appointments

The person you choose for this key role should have a good number of the following qualities:

1. **Pleasant.** Someone who is friendly and courteous can help you and your medical team feel comfortable and relaxed.

2. **Cool, calm, and collected.** You may experience a wide range of emotions before, during, and after appointments. It's helpful to have someone who stays calm and keeps his or her feelings under control.

3. **Caring.** At times you may need emotional support and encouragement from this person.

4. **Reliable.** You'll want someone who will be on time and consistently follow through.

5. **Trustworthy.** This person will see and hear a lot that must remain confidential.

6. **Respectful.** In some circumstances this person may need to step out of the room to give you and your physician privacy.

7. **Self-controlled.** Appointments are about you, not about the person with you. You need to feel confident that he or she won't try to take over a conversation or shift the focus away from you and your needs.

8. **Able to keep you on track.** If necessary, the person with you can prompt you to focus on your highest-priority questions.

9. **A good listener and clear thinker.** The person with you will need to pay close attention, ask follow-up questions if necessary, and be sure he or she understands the information shared at an appointment.

10. **A good note-taker.** Think about classmates who were great note-takers. That's the kind of note-taking you want someone doing at appointments. (See chapter 28, "Take Notes.")

Before, During, and After Your Appointment

Before each appointment, let the person know whether you'd like him or her to be primarily a silent listener and note-taker or to be more actively involved in the discussion. That may change from one appointment to the next depending on your needs. One person told me, "At most of my friend's appointments, I was mainly there to listen and take notes. Sometimes, though, he asked me to be his voice as well—asking questions and relaying information when he had trouble doing so himself."

At your appointment, introduce the person to your medical team. Explain that you'd like the team to speak as candidly as they would if they were talking only to you. As long as they know that the person has your permission to be there, there shouldn't be any problem with his or her sitting in.

One person shared his experience:

> "My wife and I agreed early on that this would be a team effort. She went to appointments with me, reminded me of what we wanted to focus on during the appointment, took notes, and communicated with medical staff to make sure we had a clear understanding of what was happening and what was needed. The staff reacted positively to her being there and included her in their conversations with me."

After the appointment, you and the other person can compare notes. You may be surprised by how much he or she caught that you didn't.

You don't need to handle your appointments alone. Having someone with you can help make the most of your time with your medical team.

28

Take Notes

"Going through a tough time like this,
I find it difficult, if not impossible,
to remember all that my oncologist tells me.
I write everything down so I won't forget anything."

All of us have had times when we were sure we'd remember something important, only to wish later that we'd written it down because the details ended up slipping out of our memory. That's a big reason why taking notes is so valuable.

Taking good notes during medical appointments will benefit you in a number of ways:

- Having notes about appointments ensures that your medical team's instructions and information about key issues, such as medications and side effects, are right at your fingertips.

- You can use your notes to share your medical team's instructions with your loved ones so they can help you most effectively.

- You can feel more confident and in control when you have access to good, detailed information from your appointments.

- Your notes help you remember answers to questions you've asked before and may suggest questions to ask in the future.

- Taking notes can strengthen your relationship with your medical team. An oncologist told me, "It's always good to see that a patient is taking notes and absorbing all he or she can. We appreciate that level of commitment."

- Taking notes helps you take a more active role in treatment.

Here's how a survivor described the importance of taking notes:

"From the day I was diagnosed, my medical team recommended that I take notes on what was said. They told me that I probably wouldn't hear or remember many of the details they shared—and they were right. Taking notes helped me ask good questions and clarify things I wasn't sure about or didn't remember."

Get the Help You Need

You may not always feel up to taking notes or organizing them. As mentioned in chapter 27, "Bring Someone with You to Appointments," one possibility is to have someone else present who can help with taking notes. When someone helps with note-taking, you're more likely to catch all the important information. Also, the other person can focus on writing down what's said, which can make it easier for you to interact with your medical team.

Your Note-Taking Approach

Find the note-taking approach that works best for you. Keep it simple and clear so you can write information down quickly and still understand it later.

Here are some guidelines that may help with your note-taking.

During the Appointment

- If you get behind in your note-taking, it's okay to ask the oncologist or other team member to repeat something.

- If you're unsure about anything, ask for clarification.

- If you hear any unfamiliar medical terms or names of medications, ask how to spell them.

- You might write down how to pronounce unfamiliar words so you can use them more comfortably in future conversations with your medical team.

After the Appointment

- Review your notes while they're still fresh in your mind. Fill in details you didn't have time to write down during the visit. It's good to do this as soon as possible after the appointment so you can better remember what you meant. Sometimes I had trouble reading my own handwriting when I didn't get back to my notes right away.

- If someone went with you to the appointment, review his or her notes as well. Discuss those notes and get clarification on anything you're unsure about. Ask whether he or she can think of any other helpful information that neither of you wrote down.

- Highlight any appointments, reminders, follow-up actions, or other tasks that need your attention.

- As you review your notes, begin a list of questions you want to ask at the next appointment.

- Some find it helpful to type their handwritten notes after the appointment or to have a friend or family member do that for them. Maintaining your notes on a computer can make them easier to read, retrieve, and search through. You can also print out any notes you want to take to a future appointment.

- Save your notes with the rest of your personal medical information. Store them in a way that makes them easy to access. Chapter 16, "Keeping Track of Personal Medical Information," gives some practical suggestions about doing this.

- You may want to review your notes as you prepare for future appointments.

In short, taking careful notes helps you be more active in your treatment and work more effectively with your medical team.

29

Focus
Your Questions

*"I kept a running list of questions that I thought
of between doctor's appointments and then put
a star by the ones I considered most pressing.
That way I was ready to ask the most important
questions at each appointment."*

Taking the time to prepare and focus your questions before meeting
with your oncologist helps ensure your appointments are as beneficial
as possible.

Medical professionals are happy to see patients give serious consideration
to what questions they ask and how they ask them. One nurse said, "Many
people become anxious the moment they get to the doctor's office. If they
don't have a list ready, they can forget to ask the most important questions.
Putting together a list of questions helps patients leave the appointment with
the information they need."

Here are six tips for focusing your questions and maximizing every
appointment with your oncologist. The first five tips are for preparing
questions *before* your appointment, while the last one is for using those
questions *during* your appointment.

1. Keep a Running List of Possible Questions

Maintain a list of questions you want to ask, adding to it whenever a new
question comes to mind. The questions in chapter 13, "Medical Questions
to Ask and When to Ask Them," can give you a number of ideas.

One person said, "I keep my smartphone by my bed, so if I think of
any questions in the middle of the night, I can record them right away."

Another said, "Have a pen and paper with you all the time because you never know when you'll think of a question."

2. Eliminate Questions That You Can Answer with Information from Other Reputable Sources

Because your time for each appointment is limited, you'll want to focus on asking questions that your oncologist can best answer. Of course, it's important to check with your oncologist about any areas of uncertainty or anything that specifically relates to your treatment, but you may be able to find answers to some of your more general questions from other reputable sources. For instance, you might:

* look up definitions in a medical dictionary (online or in print);

* find answers in printed materials your oncologist shares with you;

* obtain a list of possible side effects for a particular medication from an oncology nurse;

* get basic information about a medication from your pharmacist; or

* learn answers to general questions from the National Cancer Institute (cancer.gov or 800-422-6237), the American Cancer Society (cancer. org or 800-227-2345), or another reputable cancer organization suggested by your medical team.

Consulting such reliable sources of information in advance can conserve your appointment time for the important questions you can't find answers to elsewhere—or for questions that your oncologist can answer better than anyone else because of his or her unique perspective on you and your cancer.

3. Prioritize Your Questions before Your Appointment

Before your appointment, arrange your questions in order of importance so you can be sure to ask the most pressing questions first. Questions that can wait until later can go toward the end of the list.

4. Phrase Your Questions Clearly

Ask yourself: *What's the clearest, most concise way I can ask this question in order to get the best information?* You'll want to communicate clearly so the oncologist can know exactly what you're wondering about and can provide the most helpful answer possible.

Make sure your questions will help you obtain the information you really need. For example, a question like "What do people do for nausea?"

may be too general to get enough helpful information. It's more effective to ask a specific question that directly pertains to your own situation: "I felt nauseated the first two days after my chemotherapy. Is there something that can be done to reduce my nausea?"

Your questions don't have to be perfect, but it's good to prepare them carefully so that they're clear. It may be beneficial to have a friend or family member read them in advance and help you reword any that aren't clear or specific enough so you can get the information you're looking for.

5. Prepare Your List

Once you have your questions ready, prepare a list to take with you, including space beneath each question for your notes. If someone is going with you to your appointment, make a copy for that person.

6. At the Appointment, Ask Your Questions One by One

At the appointment, when your oncologist asks for your questions, it's best not to just hand over the list and expect him or her to read and answer them. Instead, start by asking the most important question you need answered. If you're unclear about your oncologist's answer, seek clarification and ask follow-up questions until you fully understand. Then, move on to your next question. This focused approach is much more effective at getting the answers you need.

Since the person you've brought to the appointment has a copy of your questions, he or she can help keep the discussion on track, make sure you cover the most important questions first, and take notes.

Focusing your questions certainly benefits you, but it also helps your medical team. It respects their time and expertise, and it gives them the satisfaction of being as helpful as possible to you.

30

Share Streamlined Information

"It's impossible for me to know about every study, clinical trial, and new development that might affect my patients. So it works really well when a patient who wants my thoughts about a possible new treatment gives me a concise summary."

Suppose you come across interesting information about a clinical trial, a new treatment, a different use of an existing medication, or a nonstandard therapy. After a little more searching, you find some credible articles on the subject, and you want your oncologist's thoughts. How do you share that information with him or her?

It's important *not* to hand your oncologist a stack of documents and expect him or her to read them. In the waiting room before one of Joan's appointments, I saw a patient come in with a pile of material. I overheard her saying that she was going to share with her doctor all the research she had done on a particular nonstandard therapy. The implication was that she expected her oncologist to read through all of it. That's not a helpful way to pass along information. One oncologist told me, "I've had patients bring in pages and pages of internet articles and just drop them on my desk. With everything else that comes my way each day, along with all the studying I already do to stay current, I'm not always able to do a lot of extra reading like that."

Instead, when you have information to share with your oncologist, first check its credibility (see chapter 14, "Where to Look for Information about Your Kind of Cancer"). Then try to condense it to a one-paragraph summary—or, at most, one page. Make it as concise, well organized, and easy to read as you can.

Consider using bullet points that address the following:

- What is the information about? (A new treatment? A clinical trial? A different use of an existing treatment? A nonstandard therapy?)

- What does it do? (Shrink a tumor? Relieve pain? Ease a side effect?)

- What success has it had? (What statistics are available? What scientific studies have been done on it?)

- Where has it been studied? (A hospital? A clinic? A university?)

- Where can more information be found? (A book? An article? A website?)

You may want to ask a friend or family member to read your summary to make sure it communicates clearly. Another possibility is to ask someone to help you write the summary or even to write it for you.

When you meet with your oncologist:

1. Briefly explain what you've found.

2. Offer your written summary and say that you'd like to know what your oncologist thinks.

3. Don't ask your oncologist to read all the material you've gathered, but do bring it along and mention that you have it if he or she would like to see it.

A man whose wife had cancer talked about his experience:

"When I was in the Air Force, my job was to send summary reports to the two-star general at headquarters. These reports needed to cover all the essential facts while remaining brief and to the point. If the general wanted more information, we'd provide it—as much as he wanted. But we always began with that simple one-page summary. I followed the same approach in passing along information to my wife's doctors—concise, to-the-point, get-in-and-get-out reports. I found it was exactly what they needed."

The key is to give your oncologist only as much material as he or she needs to assess the information you've found and decide how it might apply to you. When you share streamlined information, you make the most effective use of time, helping your oncologist provide you with the best possible care.

31

The Gift
of Empathy

*"My oncologist came in much later than our scheduled
appointment time, looking tired. I said, 'Tough day, huh?'
He took a deep breath, seemed to relax a bit, and said,
'Yeah. Thanks for asking.'"*

The people on your medical team serve you by helping you fight cancer.
You can serve them as well—by offering the gift of empathy.

Empathy is walking in another person's shoes. It's sensing what others
are feeling—and caring enough to mention it. Showing empathy is treating
medical professionals with kindness and respect, letting them know that you
recognize and appreciate who they are, what they do, and how hard they
work. Empathy has the power to strengthen and enrich your connection
with members of your medical team.

Empathizing can be a challenge when you're dealing with cancer. At
times it may be hard to focus on anything other than your own immediate
situation. Your medical team understands what you're experiencing and
empathizes with you. But when you are able to offer empathy to them
as well, it can make a real difference in your relationship with these key
individuals. These small caring acts can remain in team members' minds
long after your appointment.

Consider what medical professionals experience on a continuing basis.
Here's what one oncologist shared with me:

> "Oncologists face tremendous pressure every day: sick patients, life-
> threatening diagnoses, and sky-high expectations. So we definitely
> welcome empathy, especially when it's directed at our own pressure
> points, such as dismay ('Why did that happen to this person?'),

153

anxiety ('I need to get this right—have I exhausted every possibility?'), and fatigue ('I've seen a lot of complex cases today, and it's wearing me out')."

Day after day, medical professionals work with patients and family members who are frightened, impatient, angry, resigned, apathetic, sad, tired, in pain, nauseated, or any combination of these. In addition, these professionals face the daily strain of needing to make decisions that will result in the best care for each individual patient.

You can help ease these pressures by offering a little empathy in simple ways. For example:

- When your oncologist sighs while trying to reboot his computer after it froze, you could smile and say, "I hate it when something like that happens."

- When a nurse's pager goes off while she's caring for you—and then again right after that—you might say, "Sounds like it's really busy right now."

- If someone yells at the receptionist and then storms off, you can say something like, "That must be rough."

- If a medical procedure is taking longer than usual because of technical issues and the nurse seems exasperated and apologetic, you could say, "This has to be frustrating for you."

One person shared how he showed this kind of empathy:

"I was in the examination room, getting a little impatient, when my oncologist came in and apologized for the delay, saying that a couple of appointments had gone much longer than expected. As soon as I saw the look on his face, my frustration just melted away. It was clear that he'd had a long day so far caring for patients—and a good portion of the day was still ahead of him. I said, 'I guess it never gets any easier, does it?' He looked at me, smiled, and said, 'No, it really doesn't.' Just my acknowledgment seemed to pick him up a bit."

The daughter of a woman with cancer said, "My mother was just naturally empathetic with her caregivers—her oncologist, the nurses, the receptionist, and anyone else—and their relationship was that much stronger for it." A nurse told me, "We understand how hard dealing with cancer is for patients and family members, but when they show us empathy, it gives us a jolt of energy. It makes a connection that we remember."

Strengthening and enriching relationships—that's the gift of empathy.

32

Laughter Enhances the Best Medicine

"I was having a cystoscopy, and when I first looked at the screen, I gasped—I thought it was showing something terribly abnormal inside my bladder. The doctor calmly explained to me that the camera hadn't been inserted yet; it was just pointing at the floor! We had a good laugh about that, and so did the rest of my medical team when I repeated the story for them later on."

After one surgery, Joan was unable to eat normally and had to be fed intravenously for a while. When it was time for her to start eating again, she had a light meal—and immediately threw it up. We knew this meant something was wrong, and we were feeling pretty anxious.

When the surgeon came by on his rounds, his first words to Joan were, "I hear you barfed." His statement was so unexpected that it broke the tension, and we all laughed about it. Then we got right to what mattered most: how to handle the problem.

Cancer is serious business, but every now and then you might have a chance to enjoy a lighter moment with your medical team. As you can, take those opportunities and have a good laugh together. Laughter can put you and your team at ease and provide a welcome respite.

A nurse told me, "With all the stress involved in healthcare, everyone benefits from laughing together from time to time. It helps to build the bond between the patient and medical team. It increases trust and rapport. Plus, it reminds us why we got into the medical field in the first place: because we enjoy people and want to help them."

Just be sure to use humor appropriately. If the situation calls for you and the medical team to be serious, cracking a joke probably won't help. And, of course, if a joke is likely to make others uncomfortable, it would be best not to share it. But if you think the time is right for a bit of humor, go for it!

Here are some examples of lighter moments that people have shared with me.

"A Bouncing Baby Bone Marrow Sample"

"My husband went in for a bone marrow biopsy, and the doctor said I could go in with him. So he was lying on his side on the table, and I was sitting in a chair facing him. I could tell he was anxious, so I did the first thing that came to mind—the Lamaze breathing we had learned when I was pregnant with our son. My husband started doing it too, and we just kept it going, watching each other intently and doing our breathing while the doctor did the biopsy.

"Finally the doctor said, 'All done. Congratulations—you're now the proud parents of a bouncing baby bone marrow sample!' We all broke into laughter."

The Birthday Present

"After my mastectomy and chemotherapy, the plan was for me to have reconstructive surgery. The first day that would work in everyone's schedule turned out to be my birthday. I told my surgeon, 'Let's do it—I don't think anyone else will be giving me a new boob for my birthday.' He loved it!"

"Where Do You Keep the Leeches?"

"My mother and I watched a TV show about medieval medicine that described using leeches for bloodletting and putting fresh cow dung onto wounds. A few days later, we were at the pharmacy picking up her new prescription. The pharmacist explained the details about the medication and then asked, 'Do you have any questions?' My mother, who is normally very serious, said with a straight face, 'Yes, could you tell me where you keep the leeches and cow dung?' My mom and I burst into laughter. The pharmacist wasn't sure how to respond until we explained about the TV show. After that, it became our running joke; whenever we'd stop by, he'd say, 'I'm still waiting for that special order of leeches.'"

Nature Sounds

"I was having trouble falling asleep at night, so my oncologist suggested I listen to a CD that had nature sounds. At the next appointment, I mentioned that I'd bought the CD, and the doctor asked whether it helped. I said, 'Well, not really—the sound of waves kept me awake thinking about fishing, the sound of birds kept me awake thinking about hunting, and the sound of rain made me get up to pee.' The doctor couldn't keep a straight face."

The Stuffed Dog

"When my nephew was in the hospital, my family brought him a small, stuffed toy dog. Every time he went through a new procedure, we would do something to the dog—wrap it head to toe in bandages, hang a prescription bottle around its neck, put a splint on its leg, things like that. He got a real kick out of it! Whenever he hurt, we would create some new ailment for the toy dog, which helped him laugh and took his mind off the pain. When the doctors and nurses stopped by to check on him, they'd have a good laugh about the dog too. It lightened the atmosphere for everyone."

"I Don't Fly!"

"After examining my MRI, my doctor told me I needed surgery right away at a medical center 200 miles away. I heard him talking about my flying there due to the urgency. Since I'm terrified of flying, I interrupted, 'But doctor, *I don't fly!*' Without missing a beat, he looked at me and said, 'I know you don't. That's why we'll be using a helicopter.' I couldn't help but laugh. It took the edge off the situation—and, yes, I did take that helicopter ride."

The Hostess Snowball

"For my first chemotherapy treatment, I came in wearing an outlandish, fuzzy, bright-pink blouse. It was my way of showing that I wouldn't let all this scary stuff drag me down. I told the chemo nurse, 'I don't care if I look like a Hostess Snowball; I'm wearing this to every treatment!'

"The next time I went in for treatment, a nurse I didn't recognize greeted me by name when I arrived. When I asked her how she knew who I was, she said, 'You're famous around here! You're the only Hostess Snowball who comes in for chemo!' We both just had to laugh about that."

As vital as it is to take cancer seriously, it's also important to find times to laugh and share lighter moments with your medical team. That momentary break can be just what you and your team need.

33

Passivity Doesn't Work

*"I'm sort of passive by nature. In dealing with
my cancer, though, I learned early on that it
was much better for me to speak up about
my questions and needs."*

When relating and communicating with others, people can behave in three basic ways: passively, aggressively, or assertively. While you're dealing with cancer, passivity doesn't work, and neither does aggression. Only assertiveness works.

This chapter and the next two will cover each of these ways of relating. First: passivity.

What Is Passive Behavior?

Passive behavior is when people don't express their thoughts, feelings, or questions. They might avoid sharing their real needs, asking for information or clarification, or making requests. Their opinions are often easily swayed by others, and they frequently allow others to take advantage of them or make decisions for them.

What Does Passive Behavior Look Like?

Here are a couple of examples of passive behavior in interactions between people with cancer and their medical teams.

"You're the Doc"

An oncologist explained to a patient that he had at least three treatment options, each with its own advantages and disadvantages. After explaining the options, the oncologist asked, "Do you have any questions?"

The patient just shrugged.

After a pause, the oncologist asked, "Do you have any thoughts about which treatment you'd prefer?"

The patient replied, "You're the doc."

"Yes, and I want to help you any way I can, but I need to make sure you understand the options so we can make the best decision. I've explained the pluses and minuses of each of these treatments. Do you have any questions? Is there anything you aren't sure about?"

The patient shrugged again. "You know best. I'll do whatever you say."

"I'll Be Fine"

A few days after a woman had received the third of sixteen scheduled chemotherapy treatments, she and her husband went to her oncologist's office for a regularly scheduled appointment. The nurse asked, "How did you do after your recent treatment?"

The woman responded, "I did okay."

The nurse pressed the question. "Sometimes people are exhausted following this particular chemotherapy. Did you experience anything like that?"

"It was fine."

At that point, the husband shook his head and spoke up: "I'm really worried about her. I came home from work after her last treatment, and she was so weak that she couldn't get out of bed."

The nurse gently said to the woman, "If you're having difficulties with the treatment, it's important that you let us know."

The woman replied, "I just have to get through this. I have thirteen more of these, and I don't want to have to postpone them just because they wear me out."

The nurse paused before saying, "Actually, we need you to tell us what's really happening so we can help you get through all the treatments. If you don't tell us what's going on, the treatments may take so much out of you that we'll have to put them off."

The woman shook her head and said, "I'll be fine."

Why Some People May Relate Passively

People might relate passively for a number of reasons.

Sometimes people think they'll bother others if they speak up. They think it isn't worth bothering the medical team with their questions, concerns, or problems. One woman shared with me, "Mom was having a rough time during her treatments, but she told us, 'I don't want to waste the doctor's time talking about it.'"

Sometimes people misunderstand what it means to be a good patient. They believe that the best way to be a good patient is not to raise any issues or concerns.

Sometimes people assume that they don't need to communicate. They may think, *I don't need to bring it up because the doctor probably already knows about it,* or *This has probably already been communicated to everyone on the medical team.*

Sometimes people think it isn't their place to speak up with their medical team. Because they feel so awed or intimidated by medical professionals, they may believe they should quietly follow instructions and never ask any questions or raise any concerns.

Sometimes people are uncomfortable discussing certain sensitive issues. When it comes to sensitive topics such as bodily functions, potentially embarrassing physical problems, or troubling feelings or thoughts, they may talk about their situation only vaguely or not at all. One oncology nurse told me, "Sometimes patients will say, almost in a whisper, 'I don't know if I should bring this up, but . . .' and then tell me about a sensitive issue. I tell them, 'Don't be afraid to ask the doctor about that. It's a totally appropriate topic—one that comes up a lot.'"

Sometimes people don't want to show any signs of weakness. They think they should tough it out and endure silently rather than ask for help, make a request, or say anything they think could make them appear weak.

Sometimes people are afraid to speak up. They may fear possibly learning that their situation is worse than expected or worry that speaking up will result in more treatments and tests.

Sometimes people simply feel too drained to say much of anything. They may be so tired, ill, or discouraged that it's hard to muster the energy to provide information or respond to questions.

It's not uncommon to have any of these thoughts, feelings, or worries. Behaving passively, however, isn't the best way to address them.

Problems with Relating Passively

Relating passively can make things worse for both the person with cancer and his or her medical team.

The Patient May Suffer Needlessly

A nurse reflected on the suffering that passivity can cause:

> "I've seen situations where people have made things more difficult for themselves by being passive. They didn't tell us what was going on, so we thought they were doing better than they really were. As a result, we didn't make the adjustments that we could have, and the patient suffered needlessly."

The daughter of a man with cancer shared this experience:

> "When my father was in the hospital, the doctor came by and asked him how he was. Dad never wanted to be a bother, so he replied with his usual 'I'm okay.' The doctor studied the chart for a moment, then looked at Dad and said, 'With all that you've got going on, *okay* isn't the first word that comes to mind. You know, I really want to help you with any pain you're having and give you the care you need, but the only way I can do that is if you're honest with me about what you're feeling.' Dad then confessed that he'd been extremely uncomfortable the night before. The doctor changed the pain medication, and Dad's condition improved soon after."

The Medical Team May Have to Work Much Harder

A physician described the frustration of trying to communicate with passive patients:

> "If I ask, 'How have you been feeling since our last appointment?' and the patient just says, 'Fine,' I have to ask follow-up questions to get information about the patient's progress. Sometimes it's like the patient is *hinting* that something is wrong but doesn't say it, so I have to keep digging. It's always easier to focus on providing the best care when people let me know what's really going on."

An oncology nurse told me:

> "Sometimes patients are afraid to bring up important issues during an appointment. So they wait until they get home and then ask family

members, who call us, concerned and sometimes upset. We then spend time gathering more information, checking with the doctor, and getting back to them. The whole process is much easier for everyone when the patient asks these questions during the appointment."

Miscommunication, misunderstandings, missed opportunities, and misery all can result from relating passively.

Ask for Help If You Need It

Avoiding passive behavior might not come easily, especially for people who are naturally shy or who are exhausted from dealing with cancer. That's why it's good to know you can ask for help if you need it. You might ask a family member or friend to encourage you to speak up for yourself or express your needs or, in certain situations, to speak on your behalf.

An oncologist said, "I tell my patients up front, 'We can't do our job as well if you don't give us information. Speak up *early on* if you are experiencing pain, don't understand the instructions, have troublesome side effects, or sense something may be wrong. We can only treat the issues we know about, and it's much easier for you—and for us—to take care of issues right away.'"

For someone dealing with cancer, passivity doesn't work.

34

Aggression
Doesn't Work

*"While getting treatment, I'd sometimes see other
patients being harsh with their doctor or nurse.
I'd always think, 'These people are your allies!
Why slap the hands that are helping you?'"*

There may be times when cancer frays your nerves and makes you feel unusually annoyed or easily aggravated. Even though it can be tempting to lash out when that happens, treating others in aggressive ways can make matters worse.

Just as passivity doesn't work in relating with your medical team, aggression doesn't work either.

What Is Aggressive Behavior?

Aggressive behavior is when people try to get what they want at the expense of others or when they express themselves in harsh, belligerent, threatening, or hostile ways. They might make demands, manipulate people, or make decisions for others. They may label others or use put-downs, sarcasm, or profanity to intimidate people into giving them what they want.

Aggressive behavior does no one any good. Not only does it hurt those on the receiving end, but it ultimately hurts the person acting aggressively. It wastes emotional energy, damages relationships with people whose help is vital, and can be a source of embarrassment.

What Does Aggressive Behavior Look Like?

Here are some real-life examples of aggressive behavior in interactions with medical professionals.

No Rooms Available

A woman arrived with her father at his oncologist's waiting room. She interrupted the receptionist, said her father was feeling bad, and insisted that the receptionist provide a place where he could lie down. The receptionist said, "Oh, I'm so sorry. Let me find someone to help you."

A minute later, a nurse came to the waiting room, took the man's pulse, and asked him some questions. The woman harshly repeated her demand. The nurse replied, "I'm sorry, but we don't have a room available right now where your father can lie down. We'll find a place for him as soon as we can. It should only be a couple of minutes. In the meantime, I'll get him a pillow and a blanket."

As the nurse left, the woman muttered loudly enough for everyone in the waiting room to hear, "These people are totally clueless."

After a few minutes, a room opened up for her father, and the woman calmed down a little, but she continued to behave in a surly way with the staff throughout the appointment.

The Wrong Appointment Date

A man showed up at the oncologist's office and told the assistant at the check-in counter that he had an appointment for 11:30. The assistant checked her list and said, "I'm sorry, but it doesn't look like you're scheduled for an appointment today."

The man fired back, "What are you talking about? Of course I am. I wrote it down—Wednesday at 11:30. Look again; you must have missed it."

The assistant checked her computer and said a few moments later, "Our records show that your appointment is scheduled for *next* Wednesday at 11:30—a week from today. I'm sorry about the misunderstanding."

"That's wrong! You must have screwed up. I took time off work to be here, so you'd better get me in to see the doctor *today!*"

"I'm sorry for the inconvenience, sir. We can try to fit you in, but things are a little tight today, so it might be a while before the doctor can see you. I'll check and let you know what we can do."

The man glared at the assistant and snarled, "Fine!" He sat down in the waiting room, fuming.

Aggression Can Hurt the Patient's Cause

One reason not to relate aggressively is that doing so can hurt the patient's relationship with the medical team and other supporters. Responding aggressively may feel satisfying—for a minute or two—but the long-term cost of aggression can be high because it can alienate people who are providing necessary help.

An oncologist told me:

> "The husband of one of our patients turned everything into a reason to find fault. No matter what we did or said, he told us that it wasn't right or it wasn't good enough. We all wanted the same thing—to help his wife defeat the cancer—but his confrontational behavior focused much of the attention on him instead of his wife, making things more difficult for her and for us."

Another problem with aggressive relating is that it wears people out, including those who could really help the patient. A nurse shared:

> "We had a patient who constantly made unreasonable demands and berated us for the smallest things, even with our best efforts to care for her. That can really wear down a team. It's harder to keep giving your best when someone acts like that."

Aggressive behavior can damage relationships, even with people who truly want to help.

Remember the Real Enemy

It helps to remember that cancer is the real enemy and to remain focused on defeating it. The people around the patient—medical professionals, family, friends, and others who provide support along the way—are not the enemy. If a patient or loved one relates aggressively toward them, it can put a strain on those important relationships.

One man described how he handled frustration and anger as it inevitably came up:

> "Once in a while, we'd have to wait for close to an hour at the oncologist's office. Most of us took it in stride, and we'd even joke about it. But sometimes someone would get so upset they'd complain loudly to check-in personnel, nursing staff, and doctors.

> "Now, I can understand the other guy's frustration, but I also know that many times the delays were because the doctors were squeezing in other patients who had emergencies. If I were one of those emergencies, I'd definitely want them to make time for me."

Apologize, If Necessary

Anyone can get overwhelmed and behave aggressively from time to time. If you do, it's best to apologize to the other person as soon as you can. Apologizing can help you repair and rebuild your relationship with someone who is important to you so that relationship can stay strong into the future.

A nurse told me, "We understand how pain, fear, the unknown—really, everything surrounding cancer—can build up and set people off. If that happens, a heartfelt apology goes a long way."

Another, Better Way

Does avoiding aggression mean being stoic? Should you refrain from expressing your difficult feelings or being direct about your needs? Of course not.

There is a much more effective way of relating that avoids the extremes and pitfalls of both passive and aggressive behavior. That way of relating, assertiveness, is the subject of the next chapter.

35

Assertiveness Works

"I wanted to be an active part of my treatment team, so I asked lots of questions, expressed my needs to the doctor and staff, and tried to be as considerate and cooperative as possible. It really helped us appreciate and understand each other, and it helped us work well together too."

Passivity gets you nowhere, and neither does aggression. Assertiveness is what works.

What Is Assertiveness?

Some people have a mistaken idea of what assertiveness is. When they hear the word *assertiveness,* they may think of a pushy, demanding, "my way or the highway" attitude. That's not being assertive—that's just plain aggression.

Assertiveness is when people:

- stand up for their own rights as well as the rights of others;
- clearly, directly, and kindly communicate their feelings, opinions, and questions;
- are positive, respectful, and constructive as they relate to others; and
- do what they can to make sure their needs are addressed.

What Does Assertiveness Look Like?

Here are a couple of examples that medical professionals have shared with me about patients relating assertively.

"How Have You Been Doing?"

The oncologist entered his office and sat down across from his patient. "So, how have you been doing since you last came in?" he asked.

The man said, "Honestly, it's been a rough week. I've been having nausea more frequently, and it's been difficult to deal with."

"Tell me more about what's been happening," the oncologist said. "We should be able to help you out with that."

The man gave the details about what he'd experienced, adding, "Also, the nausea medicine doesn't seem to be working well for me. I usually start feeling nauseated again not that long after I take it."

The oncologist asked some additional questions, looked over his past notes, and said, "I think we can find a better solution."

"Could I Get an Appointment Earlier in the Morning?"

A woman had finished her treatment. Her oncologist told her that the treatment had been successful, and there was no evidence of cancer remaining. He asked her to come back in a specific number of months for a checkup.

After the appointment, she went to the receptionist and told her, "Good news—no sign of cancer! I don't need to come back again until August."

The receptionist said, "Congratulations, that's great to hear!" She then checked the computer. "Okay, how about Monday the 5th at 2:00 in the afternoon?"

The woman replied, "Actually, an afternoon appointment wouldn't fit my work schedule. Could I get a morning appointment instead?"

"Sure. I'll see what's available." After checking the computer again, the receptionist said, "How about Tuesday the 6th at 10:30 A.M.—would that work?"

The woman thought it over a bit before saying, "A 10:30 appointment *could* work, but something earlier would work even better. Do you happen to have anything earlier than that?"

The receptionist checked the schedule again and said, "Nothing earlier on the 6th. But on the following day, Wednesday the 7th, we have an opening at 9:00. How about that?"

The woman nodded and smiled. "That would work great. Thank you so much for checking."

Assertiveness Builds Relationships

Assertiveness—open, honest, and collaborative communicating and relating—builds positive relationships with your medical team and others around you. It reduces tension, increases trust, and enhances the flow of information, leading to better decisions and more effective care.

A nurse explained, "The patient is the most important person on the team. Without the patient, there's no reason for the team to exist. His or her needs, wants, and expectations are what matter most. So it really helps when patients let us know exactly what they're thinking."

Another nurse said, "We have the same goal as the patient: to defeat the cancer. When the patient communicates and relates assertively, it helps us work together to achieve that goal."

Being assertive is a great way to ensure that people on your medical team look forward to working with you. One physician told me, "Without a doubt, working with assertive patients is most gratifying, professionally and personally."

How to Be an Assertive Patient

For some people, assertiveness comes easily. For others who aren't used to relating in this way, it can take some effort, but it is possible to grow in this area. Here are some tips for assertive communication with your medical team—all based on what physicians, nurses, and other medical professionals have said.

Be Informed about and Involved in Your Medical Care

Assertive patients are informed and involved. A physician said, "It's great to work with patients who are eager to know what's going on and who actively participate in decision making."

Be Prepared to Talk with Your Medical Team

Your appointments will go more smoothly when you come prepared to talk with your medical team about what's most important to you.

A nurse gave this description: "Well-prepared patients are specific. They come in having already thought about what they want to discuss. That helps them be calmer, clearer, and more logical with their questions. Then, when they get an answer, they move on to the next question. They make sure they don't leave with any questions unanswered."

Answer Questions Clearly and Honestly

You can help your medical team gather the complete information they need by answering their questions clearly, honestly, and directly.

A physician said:

"When I ask patients how they've been doing since I last saw them, some just give a one- or two-word answer, and then I have to work a lot harder to learn the necessary details. But other patients say more right off the bat. They might say something like 'Here's what's going well,' or 'Here's what isn't going so well,' and they describe exactly what they're experiencing. When a patient communicates like that, it helps us both."

Take Responsibility for Communication

Assertive patients take responsibility for making sure that necessary communication takes place. Here's how a physician's assistant described the benefits of working with patients who relate this way:

"When they have a concern, they bring it up. They get right to the point with statements and questions like 'This is what's bothering me. Is there something we can do about it?' That makes each office visit a lot more productive. Not only can we answer their questions, but we can quickly determine what their needs are and how best to meet them."

Ask Questions

A big part of communicating assertively is asking questions. Ask about anything and everything you need to know.

A person with cancer told me:

"Physicians can't answer questions you don't ask. If you're uncertain about anything, ask. If you don't understand the initial answer, ask for clarification. Physicians expect you to ask questions, and they can provide even better care for you when you do. My oncologist made it clear to me from the beginning: 'There's no such thing as a dumb question.' I appreciated her saying that."

A physician told me she offers this reassurance to patients: "You never need to be apologetic about asking questions. You're the one being treated, so you can ask anything, and we'll be happy to answer."

See chapter 29, "Focus Your Questions," for ways to get the most out of your opportunities to ask questions.

After You Ask, Listen

After stating your needs, concerns, or questions, give the physician or other medical professional a chance to respond, and listen carefully to what he or she says. Listening opens the door for two-way communication and helps prevent misinformation or misunderstandings. A nurse said, "Staff really appreciate it when patients ask questions and then listen. It tells us that they want to understand what's going on and be fully involved in the treatment process."

Ask Your Oncologist about What You Find in Your Research

If your research turns up something of interest, such as a clinical trial or a newly developed treatment, ask your oncologist about it. Your assertive inquiry may open up new possibilities for you. See chapter 30, "Share Streamlined Information," for thoughts on how to talk about this kind of information with your oncologist.

Be as Relaxed and Confident as Possible in Your Relating

Medical team members feel comfortable around assertive patients because such patients relate in a calm, confident manner. Although this can be difficult while dealing with cancer, assertive patients do their best to keep their emotional reactions from getting in the way.

A physician reflected on the pleasure of relating with assertive patients:

> "When people are assertive, they present very clear concerns, questions, or issues that they want to discuss, without getting too intense about it. It's just, 'This is what I'm dealing with this week,' and 'This is what I've heard,' and 'Here are some questions I have. What do you think?' Their relaxed, open attitude sets the stage for a more meaningful conversation."

Be Courageous

It takes courage to fight cancer—chapter 39, "Praise Yourself for Your Courage," says more about that. But at times people may mistakenly think that being courageous means looking strong, enduring pain, denying fatigue, and keeping their thoughts and feelings bottled up instead of assertively speaking up about what they're experiencing. In other words, they sometimes think that being courageous means not being assertive.

Actually, one of the best ways you can manifest courage is to relate assertively—to acknowledge pain or fatigue, ask questions, express feelings, request help, and communicate needs and concerns honestly and directly. I encourage you to be courageous and practice assertiveness.

The Benefits of Assertiveness

Assertiveness has important benefits over passive or aggressive communicating and relating.

You'll build better relationships. Assertive relating is respectful, and mutual respect leads to good relationships.

You'll engage in clearer communication. Assertive communication helps your medical team better understand your specific needs and wants, and it helps you become much better informed about your cancer and treatment options.

You'll feel better about yourself. Assertiveness helps you feel more connected to other people, better cared for, and more in control.

You and your medical team will work together more effectively. Your assertive communicating and relating helps your medical team provide you with the care and support you need.

In short, assertiveness works.

36

Be an
Appreciator

"Our family wanted to show some extra appreciation to Mom's medical team. We thought it would be fun to include them in our family's annual 'Christmas in July' cookie exchange—except that the staff wouldn't have to bring anything; they'd just get cookies from us. We brought in a big platter of treats with a note from Mom. They were delighted to be part of our celebration and to know how much they meant to us."

Suppose you're on vacation and a good friend is watching your house for you—collecting the mail, walking and feeding your dog, mowing the lawn. You'll probably send that friend a card to express your thanks. You might even pick up a gift for him or her, perhaps something unique to the area where you're vacationing.

You may want to show that same sort of appreciation for your medical team. Treat them the way you would treat your good friends when they help you. When you let the people on your medical team know how much their care means to you, it can have a real impact on your relationship with them.

Your Words Can Show Appreciation

You don't need to spend a lot of money to show your appreciation. Your words, spoken or written, are often enough to let people on your medical team know that you're grateful for their care. An oncology nurse said, "Patients come in for some very unpleasant treatments, but as they leave, they'll sometimes smile and say, 'That treatment was a real pain, but you're always so kind. Thank you.' Those folks really tug at my heart!"

An oncologist told me what a simple card means to her: "When a patient writes me a personal note, it's the most precious gift. It's really special because it comes from the heart, showing that I helped him or her feel better." A nurse said, "A card makes me feel good about what I do and helps me through the tougher days."

One woman shared, "I wrote thank-you notes to my surgeon and medical team. My husband is a pediatrician, and I know how much he appreciates cards or any kind of written thanks. It means a lot when patients acknowledge what their medical team does for them."

Doing a Little More

Sometimes you may want to do more. If you go on a vacation, for instance, you might send your medical team a postcard saying something like "I couldn't be enjoying this trip without all you've done for me!" If you know your oncologist likes wine, you might bring a special bottle as a gift. Or one day you could bring snacks to your oncologist's office for the team to enjoy.

Show appreciation in ways that are within your means and that you feel comfortable doing. Here are a couple of ideas that medical professionals have said meant a lot to them.

Provide Official Recognition

When your medical team does an excellent job, you may want to recognize them officially by letting the hospital or medical center administration know about the high level of care your team gave you. Team members will feel appreciated, and your recognition will show their employers what a good job they're doing. An oncology nurse described what this meant to her:

> "Our medical center has a program where patients can recommend members of their medical team for the Guardian Angel Award. A patient did that for me, and that meant more than anything. I know intellectually that I'm making a difference, but getting that kind of official recognition helped me realize that on a more personal level."

Another nurse said:

> "Occasionally patients will write a letter to the hospital, commending their medical team for providing excellent, compassionate care. They may mention specifics that were especially important to them. It doesn't happen very often, but it's a great way for patients to show appreciation."

Find Out What They Would Like

A good way to show appreciation is to learn what the person would really enjoy and then offer it to him or her. Sometimes you can find this out just by paying attention. A man shared this story:

> "When I was in for chemotherapy, I'd sometimes overhear the nurses talking. The nurse who always cared for me was really excited that her oldest child was going to Duke University that fall. One day I stopped by the sporting goods store and bought her a baseball cap with the Duke logo on it. When I gave it to her, she teared up and said, 'You heard me talking about my son. Thank you—this means a lot to me, and my son will love seeing me wear it!'"

You also might simply ask what they would like. A receptionist told me, "Some of our staff are on special diets or have food allergies, so it's especially nice when patients ask what we'd like before they bring food for the office staff."

A Few Important Considerations

As I talked to medical professionals about their experiences with patients showing appreciation, they suggested a few important points to keep in mind.

Respect professional boundaries. Most medical professionals want to keep their relationships with patients and families professional rather than social. Be sensitive to these kinds of boundaries. For instance, it might cross the line to offer to take your oncologist and his or her spouse out to dinner, but giving them a gift certificate for a restaurant may be appropriate.

Don't give gifts that add to the team's responsibilities. If a gift comes with requirements attached, it's probably better to think of something else. An oncology nurse said, "I'd rather a patient didn't give us a plant, because then we have to take care of it. And if it wilts, everyone will feel terrible." Make sure the gift doesn't put any pressure on your medical team; you want to help them feel good, not add another task to their day.

Consider giving something the entire team can enjoy. It's perfectly appropriate to give a gift to a specific medical professional who's helped you a lot, but it can also be good to acknowledge your team as a whole and give something they all can enjoy. A basket of snacks or a thank-you card addressed to the team, for example, can brighten the day of all the people who are working with you.

If in doubt, ask. Hospitals, clinics, and other institutions often have guidelines or policies about gifts. If you're wondering whether a gift would be appropriate, just ask.

How Being an Appreciator Makes a Difference

Being an appreciator warms people's hearts. A physician described it this way:

> "As a professional and a human being, it's nice to be appreciated. We went into medicine because we want to help people, but we deal with a lot of stress in healthcare, and that can take a toll on our outlook and feeling of job satisfaction. When we hear that we really are helping, it can lift us right up—it lets us know that we're fulfilling the goal that got us started in this field."

Your acts of appreciation also strengthen your relationship with your medical team. A nurse said, "When patients show appreciation, it makes them memorable. You realize that these patients see you as a real person and truly value what you're doing."

An act of care and affirmation makes a lasting impression. When I met with one oncologist, he opened a file drawer and told me, "I've kept every card or note that patients have sent me. I have 25 years' worth at this point. Sometimes I pull out a file and read through a few of the notes. It reminds me why I do what I do." A nurse I spoke with keeps the cards and notes she receives on a bulletin board. "It's close to overflowing now," she said. "Seeing all those expressions of thanks helps me recognize the difference we've been making in people's lives—and it reenergizes me to continue."

Your grateful words and acts of kindness remind everyone on your medical team how important they are and how valuable their work is. Such appreciation builds a closer, stronger relationship with those who work so hard on your behalf.

37

Help Your Medical Team Help You

"This was a battle for my life, and I was counting on a team of well-trained and highly skilled professionals—but I knew I had to do my part too. I decided to be the best patient I could be and help any way I could."

In the movie *Jerry Maguire,* the title character is a sports agent trying to negotiate a new contract for professional football player Rod Tidwell. As the story progresses, Maguire grows increasingly frustrated with Tidwell, whose behavior keeps getting in the way of the negotiations. In a pivotal scene, an exasperated Maguire asks Tidwell to tone down his attitude, saying, "Help *me* help *you.*"

Your medical team wants to help you; their goal is to provide you with the best care possible. Your actions and behaviors, as well as those of your loved ones, can either support them or hinder them in achieving that goal. This chapter draws on principles from earlier chapters to identify specific ways you can help your medical team help you.

Seven Ways *Not* to Relate to Your Medical Team

Sometimes the best way to recognize what to do in a particular situation is to start by looking at what not to do. So here are seven ways not to relate to the medical team. Medical personnel have told me that they've encountered all these behaviors from time to time.

1. **Don't hold back information.** Oncologist after oncologist and nurse after nurse told me this essential point: Patients need to communicate fully about what they're thinking, feeling, and experiencing.

   Be honest and open with your medical team. Don't refrain from saying something because you're too embarrassed, afraid you'll sound stupid, or worried that you'll bother your medical team. If you have a question or concern, or if you think you're experiencing a symptom or side effect, let them know. You help them do their job by telling them everything that's going on with you.

2. **Don't use time ineffectively—yours or your medical team's.** Your medical team wants to provide the best possible care for you and all their other patients. Because they have only so many hours each day to interact with patients, time is a precious commodity for everyone.

   It's to your benefit to make the most efficient and effective use of your time with your medical team. That's why it's so helpful to prepare for appointments—for example, by writing down questions or concerns, bringing along a list of medications you're taking, or keeping a log of how you're feeling. Spending even a little time preparing for an appointment will help you get the most out of your time with your medical team.

3. **Don't ignore your role in working with the team.** You can count on your medical team to help you in many ways. At the same time, however, it's important to remember your responsibility for understanding your treatment plan and helping to make decisions along the way.

   When someone on your medical team gives you a choice or asks your opinion, he or she really does want to know what you think and what you want. You are a key contributor in the decision-making process. Ask any questions necessary to understand your options, and then let your medical team know what you're thinking.

   If these responsibilities sound challenging, remember that you don't have to bear them alone. Your loved ones and your medical team stand ready to help you.

4. **Don't neglect your treatment plan.** Your medical team will work with you to come up with the best possible treatment plan, but for the plan to be effective, you need to follow the team's instructions and recommendations. Of course, say something if your treatment seems to be causing major or unexpected side effects or an adverse reaction. But instead of making

changes to the plan on your own, contact your medical team and work with them to address any problems or questions that arise.

5. **Don't expect your medical team to be superheroes.** In some ways, the people on your medical team *are* like superheroes. They are highly trained, intelligent, committed individuals who regularly save lives. But they're still human. They get tired, they have physical limitations, they feel sad or frustrated at times, and they can wear down under the pressures of a demanding, difficult job.

It's important to keep your expectations realistic. Members of your medical team won't know everything and may not always act exactly as you'd like. However, they'll do everything humanly possible to help you.

6. **Don't lash out.** Admittedly, this can be tough. There may be times when you feel awful, when all the news seems bad, when you're exhausted, or when your anxiety or frustration level is through the roof. It might not be easy to keep your temper in check on such days.

It's certainly all right to let your difficult feelings out, as described in chapter 7, "Accept and Express Your Feelings," but do your best not to lash out at your medical team with those feelings. Remember that the people on the team are all on your side. An oncologist told me:

> "It's only natural for patients or family members to be upset, frustrated, or disappointed at times, and it's okay to express those feelings. I know the toll cancer can take. But we're here to help patients, so don't push us away or shut the door on communication. We need to keep the dialogue open and work together."

7. **Don't be the patient or family member from hell.** Nobody is at his or her best when dealing with cancer, and medical professionals have a great deal of understanding and sympathy for what patients and their loved ones are experiencing. However, the more consistently kind you are with your team, the stronger your relationship with them will be.

Seven Helpful Ways *to* Relate to Your Medical Team

With those seven hindrances in mind, here are seven helpful ways to relate to your medical team.

1. **Communicate openly and honestly.**

2. **Respect your team's knowledge and commitment.**

3. Take personal responsibility.

4. Relate assertively—not passively or aggressively.

5. Have realistic expectations of your team.

6. Relate compassionately to team members as fellow human beings.

7. As you can, smile.

Keep communicating with your medical team. Above all, show them the same kindness, patience, and courtesy that you'd like them to have for you.

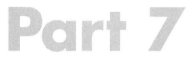

Part 7

Defining and Caring for Yourself

38

Don't Let Cancer Define You

"You may have cancer, but cancer doesn't need to have you. I took the time I needed for treatments and healing, but I lived my life as normally as possible. My life wasn't all about cancer."

Cancer changes your life, without a doubt. However, you don't have to let it control your life.

Admittedly, it can sometimes be hard to keep cancer from consuming every waking thought, especially soon after the diagnosis. At times, it may be the only thing on your mind. Doctor appointments, lab tests, treatments, side effects—everything seems to revolve around cancer.

But in spite of all this, you are still you. Cancer hasn't changed that. It's just one part of your life right now, not the whole of it. Even though it greatly affects you, it doesn't have to define you. *You* define you.

I've talked with people who have found a number of ways to keep cancer from defining them. Their thoughts and suggestions may point toward other possibilities for you.

Keep Up Your Routine as You Can

Some survivors and loved ones find routine to be comforting; it keeps them grounded when other areas of life seem out of control. Although they might need to adjust some parts of their routine, it's reassuring for them to maintain their usual activities as much as possible. One person shared:

"Life went on after my diagnosis, and so did I. When I felt up to taking the kids to school or sports practices, I kept that part of my routine, and when I didn't, my husband would do it. When I felt like it, I would cook, meet my friends for coffee, or even do some yard work. Doing my normal activities, when I could, kept me feeling normal."

Another said:

"Before cancer, I went out almost daily for a walk. Doing so grounded me and gave me time for quiet contemplation. After the diagnosis, I was determined to keep it up—I didn't want to let cancer take that time away from me. I was still able to get outside almost every day, and I enjoyed every minute of it!"

Adapt to Changes That Cancer Brings

Some people have defined themselves by adapting to the changes brought on by cancer. One man told me:

"I always enjoyed water skiing. After the cancer treatment, though, I couldn't maintain my balance on the skis like I used to. A friend suggested I try wakeboarding. He said it took a completely different stance from water skiing, and it might be more manageable for me. I tried it, and he was right. So I was able to learn a new sport and keep cancer from taking away a big part of my life."

A woman shared:

"My job was important to me, but I didn't have the energy to put in a full work week during treatment. I worked out a reduced work schedule so I would have extra time to rest and recover. Being able to keep working kept me sane; during those hours in my office, cancer was the farthest thing from my mind."

You might not be able to do everything exactly as you used to, but there may be ways to adapt and keep enjoying what's meaningful to you.

Choose Your Focus

I've talked to people who found it helpful to keep cancer from being their only focus. They decided there were other things in their lives more important than cancer, and they did their best to focus on those areas when possible instead of letting cancer consume all their time and attention.

The wife of a survivor shared this insight: "My husband said cancer was like the hum of a refrigerator. If we gave it too much attention, it might be all we could hear. So we chose to listen to other things in life. We didn't want the cancer to be the only thing we heard."

Another person put it this way: "Focus on something that makes you smile. Whether it's a hobby, your job, traveling, or something else, concentrate on that as much as you can."

A woman told me about a way she would shift the focus off cancer from time to time:

> "When I was feeling well enough to get out of the house, my friend would come over to give me a ride. As we left the house, when I was shutting the door behind me, I would say I was slamming the door on cancer and telling it to stay home while we went out to have fun. Those were some of the most rewarding times for me."

Talk about Something Else

Sometimes survivors and their families need to talk about cancer, and sometimes they need to talk about something else—to let other aspects of their lives get the attention they deserve. Focusing on those other topics is one way people can keep cancer from defining them.

A teacher who had cancer told me:

> "When my department chair came to visit, we'd talk about the department—and only a little about my illness. Since I'm one of the most experienced teachers, he continued to seek my advice about a number of issues. It was a great gift to talk about something besides cancer. It helped me feel human."

A person going through treatment said:

> "I've let my friend know that cancer doesn't always need to be at the top of our list of discussion topics. We do talk about it, but when I feel like I've said enough about cancer for the time being, we'll set that aside and chat about our children, our hobbies, or something else that's fun and rewarding."

Do What Gives Your Life Meaning

Some people said they defined themselves by becoming involved in activities that gave their lives meaning. A woman diagnosed with breast cancer attended a Stephen Series Leader's Training Course[1] where I was teaching. She told me:

---

1 For information about the Stephen Series, go to stephenministries.org.

"One way I'm standing up to cancer is by being here. When our church asked me to attend this event to learn how to help lead our Stephen Ministry, I decided: *You know what? I'm going to do this, and I'm not going to let cancer control what I'm doing or what choices I make in life.* Caring ministry is something I feel called to do, so here I am."

Being part of something bigger than yourself—something that's important to you—can push cancer out of the spotlight for a while.

As Much as Possible, Keep Doing What You Enjoy

A number of people I talked with defined themselves by continuing, as much as possible, to do the activities they truly enjoyed. They decided cancer would not take their joy away.

One woman shared, "My grandfather loves to play tennis and doesn't see any reason to give it up just because he has cancer, even if it means playing less often than before. He just figures that since playing makes him happier, it's good to keep it up whenever he can."

Try Something New

A good way to keep cancer from taking control is to try out some new experiences. If you enjoy listening to music, try a new artist or genre. If you like cooking, try a new recipe or cuisine. If you like learning, take a class. Find something new that you think you'd enjoy—and that you have the energy for—and give it a try.

One person said, "I enrolled in an astronomy class so I could focus on something much larger than my cancer: the cosmos! Studying the night sky and discussing the vastness of the universe gave me a new perspective on life."

Continue to Be Who You Are

Cancer may hurt you, it may limit you, it may thrust unwelcome changes upon you—but it doesn't define you. One daughter told me about her mother's response to cancer:

"For Mom, it's always been about family, and she isn't about to let cancer rob her of that. She's always talking about her grandchildren, the ones already born and the ones still on the way. As an avid knitter, she continues to make blankets, hats, sweaters, and scarves for her grandchildren. It's her way of not letting it be all about the cancer."

A survivor said, "Cancer has not defined me. When I had cancer, I deliberately decided that I was not going to let it take over. I kept telling myself: *There's more to me than cancer.* The cancer was an event in my life, but it is not my life."

You may find a variety of ways to resist cancer's intrusion into your life. Whatever works for you, I encourage you to do it and to hold on to who you are. Don't let cancer define you.

39

Praise Yourself for Your Courage

*"People told me I was courageous, but I didn't see myself that way. I was just doing what I needed to do to fight the cancer and continue life with my family. But as I look back, I think **anybody** dealing with cancer is courageous."*

As someone facing cancer, you are truly courageous.

That may seem like a bold statement. You might think, *What, me? No way—I'm terrified! I'm the last person you'd call courageous.*

But whatever you may think right now, you're showing a lot of courage just by doing what you can in the face of cancer. You've earned the right to praise yourself for your courage.

Cancer patients often say they don't see themselves as courageous. One person told me, "I'm really not all that courageous. I'm only going to treatments, dealing with cancer, and living my life."

But that's the epitome of courage. By getting up each morning, learning what you can, working with your medical team, dealing with treatments—plus carrying on with daily life—you are exhibiting real courage.

One reason people sometimes downplay their courage is because they equate *courageous* with *fearless,* and they've certainly felt fearful. But as Mark Twain once wrote, "Courage is resistance to fear, mastery of fear—not absence of fear."[1] Courageous people do what needs to be done in spite of their fear. That's a perfect description of someone who is facing cancer—or of a loved one supporting a person with cancer.

When you're first diagnosed, cancer can knock you off your feet. Just getting back up again and asking, *Okay, what do I do now?* is courageous.

---

1 Mark Twain, *Pudd'nhead Wilson* (New York: P.F. Collier & Son, 1894, 1899, 1922), p. 101.

As one person said, "I was scared, but I decided to do what was necessary to retake control of my life."

Going through treatment is courageous. Surgery, chemotherapy, radiation—it takes guts and determination to deal with any cancer treatment. A survivor told me, "I showed up each time for radiation even though it was the last thing I wanted to do. You do what you have to do."

Cancer may mean dealing with significant changes to your body, your emotions, and how you see your future. Coming to grips with these changes takes courage. A man I spoke to said, "Knowing how I looked after treatment, it took me a while to start going out again instead of hiding at home. But eventually I got up and got on with my life."

Continuing your daily life as you're able is also an exercise in courage. When cancer becomes a major focal point, it can be difficult to keep your life in balance. One woman told me, "During my treatment, I put every bit of strength into caring for my children. It was difficult, but I wanted to maintain some normalcy in their lives." That's courage.

Being courageous doesn't mean toughing it out alone—it takes courage to turn to others. A man shared, "My daughter prided herself on being strong and independent. But she knew that during her treatment, she needed support for her and her kids, so she found the courage to ask me for help." (See chapter 46, "Accept Help," for more thoughts about this.)

For those of you walking alongside someone with cancer: You are courageous too. You're standing by your loved one and possibly doing things you never thought you could do. One woman said, "All the times I took Mom to treatments, cared for her, or just sat with her, I never really thought of it as courage. I just saw myself as trying to do what was best for her." By hanging in there and doing what you can, you are showing tremendous courage.

It's healthy and good for your morale to recognize and affirm your courage. I'm not saying to go around telling the world how courageous you are, but it wouldn't hurt to give yourself a pat on the back every once in a while.

You deserve it. You *are* courageous.

40

Do Something Nice for Yourself

*"I kept a list on my refrigerator of fun things I
wanted to do. Then, when I felt up to it, I'd pick one
and do it. It gave me something to look forward to
and ways I could treat myself now and then."*

It's important to find ways to do something nice for yourself—actually, to do many nice things for yourself.

The challenges of cancer can take a lot out of you, so treat yourself to enjoyable experiences when you can. This can give you a healthy boost and make it a little easier to keep going.

A friend of mine whose wife had cancer decided that they could get away from it all for a little while. They traveled to a bed and breakfast and spent a long weekend enjoying the fall foliage and visiting antique shops, wineries, and a local fair. It was a great time for both of them.

Such a trip might not be practical or doable for everyone, but it demonstrates a key idea: When it comes to doing something nice for yourself, don't hold back. Do what you really want to do whenever you can. It will give you a much-needed, well-deserved break from dealing with cancer.

You can probably come up with all sorts of ways to do something nice for yourself. They don't have to be extravagant—even simple things you enjoy doing can work wonders. Here are some ideas, ranging from no cost to a larger cost.

Of course, check with your medical team if you have any questions about doing any of these activities.

For No Cost

You can do something nice for yourself in lots of ways that don't cost anything. Go for these free activities whenever you feel like it—they can be "a nice little vacation from cancer," as one person called it. Here are a number of things people have told me they've done:

- Go on a picnic at the park or in your backyard.
- Listen to some of your favorite music.
- Watch some funny videos online.
- Play a musical instrument.
- Play a card or board game with family and friends.
- Go for a walk.
- Read a book that you have on your shelf but haven't gotten to yet, or reread a book you love.
- Join a free fantasy sports league.
- Watch a favorite movie.
- Relax with a loved one in front of the fireplace.
- Visit family or friends in person or via video chat.
- Go to a free concert in the park.
- Tend your garden.
- Have a cup of coffee at home with a friend.
- Watch a sunset or sunrise.

For a Small Cost

Other activities are inexpensive enough that you can probably do them fairly often. Spending a bit of money on yourself in this way can feel good. People I've talked with have suggested ideas like these:

- Stroll through a zoo or nature park, or just sit and watch the animals.
- Visit a museum, botanical garden, or other attraction.
- Do something creative like painting, sewing, or woodworking.
- Take a drive in the countryside or to a spot that you find beautiful and relaxing.
- Go fishing.
- See a movie at a theater, or rent one to watch at home.

- Play a round of miniature golf.
- Get a new game for your mobile device.
- Pick up some snacks that you enjoy.
- Make one of your favorite meals or desserts and then eat it by candlelight.
- During the holidays, drive around to see the Christmas lights.
- Go shopping—window-shopping or browsing an online store costs you nothing, and if you find something you really like and can afford, you might go ahead and buy it.
- Buy a new book, movie, or music album.
- Catch a dramatic or musical performance at a school or community theater.
- Build a model car or airplane.
- Get a pedicure or a manicure.
- Subscribe to an online movie or TV service.
- Purchase a flowering plant or a bouquet of flowers.
- Stop by your favorite coffeehouse or ice cream shop to treat yourself.

For a Larger Cost

Occasionally it might be worth it to spend more money, as you are able, on something nice for yourself—maybe as a special reward for finishing a round of treatment, for example. Here are ideas people have shared with me:

- Go out for a nice dinner at a favorite restaurant.
- Splurge on a bottle of wine that you really enjoy.
- Attend a concert, play, or musical.
- Get a new electronic gadget.
- Start a collection of something that interests you, or add to a current collection.
- Buy some artwork that catches your eye.
- Attend a major sporting event.
- Get a massage or a facial, or spend an entire day at a spa.
- Take a vacation somewhere you've always wanted to visit.
- Go on a cruise.

These are just a few suggestions to get you started. Think about what you'd really like to do—and then do it.

As you can, give yourself breaks to indulge in the things you enjoy. Little luxuries now and then can make a big difference in how you feel.

41

Go Easy on Yourself

"I was in church one Sunday after a particularly rough treatment. I tried to stand up for a hymn, but I was having a real hard time of it. An older woman behind me tapped my shoulder and whispered, 'It's all right to sit.' Her kind words stuck with me—she gave me permission to give myself a break."

Cancer can change what you're able to do—at least for a time. You probably won't be able to carry as full a load or multitask as you did before. You may tire more easily and have trouble tackling certain chores. You might not be able to work as much. You might find your emotions are more intense at times, and little things may get to you more easily.

With such changes, it's easy to get frustrated with your limitations, but it's not worth beating yourself up over them. You have more than enough stress to deal with. Don't add to it by getting down on yourself.

Instead, go easy on yourself.

A survivor shared his experience:

"I was raised to work hard and not ask for help, even when I was under the weather. I thought that if I slowed down, I'd be letting the family down. But over time I realized that I couldn't do it all—asking someone for help or taking a nap now and then was okay. Once I stopped pushing myself so hard and getting angry with myself when I didn't measure up, I had more energy for what was really important."

Going easy on yourself involves setting realistic expectations. Discover what you can and can't do—or perhaps what isn't as easy for you as it used to be—and then do what you can. As one person said, "I just learned to accept my limitations without guilt."

One woman described it like this: "While I was going through treatment, I didn't have any extra energy. My body would say it was done for the day, and that meant it was done—I just hoped that I could make it to the couch! So I didn't push myself. I learned to listen to my body, slow down when I needed to, and be at peace with those things I just couldn't get done."

You can also ask your family and friends to assist you or even take on some of your responsibilities for a while. One person said, "My wife was more than happy to take on tasks that I wasn't up to. She'd mow the lawn and get the bills paid while I rested. I was grateful for her support in doing what needed to be done." Another shared, "During chemo, I was too weak to stand at the stove to cook, so I got my kids involved. I'd teach them while sitting on a stool by the stove. It was an opportunity to introduce them to cooking, and they had a lot of fun while helping me out."

You may find it helpful to sit down and rest now and then during your daily activities. Take breaks whenever you need them. A survivor told me, "I got tired easily, so I took things one step at a time. I'd break up tasks into small chunks; I'd do what I could, then give myself a mini-break to read or take a nap, and then work on the next step. It gave me at least some control, even if I had to take things more slowly."

You may even come up with some creative solutions for activities you'd like to do but can't. A father with cancer shared what he did:

> "At first I was frustrated with myself because I'd lost the energy I once had. It especially bothered me that I couldn't keep up with my children or be there for some of their school activities. But rather than dwell on what I *couldn't* do, I focused on what I *could* do. I asked my family to make videos of a couple of school events that I wasn't able to attend. Then we watched them together as a family, and my children had fun telling me about what was happening."

As one person put it, "When you have cancer, it's not selfish to focus more on yourself, put your own needs first, and ask others to do some things for you. In fact, I've learned that it's absolutely necessary." It's okay to go easy on yourself. When you accept what you can't do and focus on what you can do, you make your life a lot easier.

42

Holidays and Other Celebrations

"I love hosting Thanksgiving dinner. It's a family tradition. But when I had cancer, I just wasn't up to it. So several family members came over and did the cleaning, preparation, and cooking for me. I mostly rested, pitching in as I could. We all chatted and laughed. It was nice to maintain the tradition."

For many, holidays are steeped in tradition. They can be times to gather with family and friends, to share old memories and make new ones.

But cancer can change how you think about and experience holidays. You may notice this most during November to January, with the rapid succession of holidays from Thanksgiving to New Year's—but it also can be true for any other holiday, celebration, or occasion that's special to you.

Types of Changes

Cancer can change what you're *physically* able to do. With cancer treatment, you might not have the energy to prepare for holidays or participate the way you're used to. It may be difficult or impossible to travel to visit family or friends. Limitations like these can be frustrating.

Cancer also affects how you experience holidays *emotionally*. During holidays, any difficult feelings you're dealing with can be amplified. You may be thinking, *What is there to be happy about this year? I'm feeling miserable because of this cancer, and holidays are just making it worse.* When everyone around you is enjoying a holiday and you aren't, it can be hard to take.

Cancer can change holidays *financially* as well. Your budget might already be strained because of the cancer, leaving you with less to spend on gifts, decorations, meals, or other activities.

Ways to Make the Most of Holidays

Even if holidays aren't the same as they were in the past, they still can bring you joy and comfort. Here are some thoughts about how to make the most of holidays and other celebrations.

Communicate with others beforehand. Take the guesswork out of it—let family members know about your limitations, expectations, and desires. One survivor said, "As my birthday approached, I told my family ahead of time what I wanted and how much I felt up to doing. They were very understanding and planned a nice, quiet celebration."

Keep some traditions. If traditions give you a lot of comfort and enjoyment, keep as many of them as you can, or change them just enough to make things easier for you. For instance, if you can't imagine Christmas without seeing the house decked out with lights, wreaths, a Christmas tree, and Nativity scenes, then go for it—while getting help as needed so you don't exhaust yourself.

Drop or change some traditions. It's all right if you don't do everything you normally would to celebrate. Skip the Memorial Day cookout in the park and perhaps just grill in your backyard. If you don't feel up to staying awake until midnight to ring in the New Year, don't push yourself; you can count down to midnight in an earlier time zone and then go to bed. Drop or change traditions however you need to. One man said, "My wife and I would always go out to dinner at the same restaurant on Valentine's Day. But the year she was in chemo, we ate a simple meal at home by candlelight. It was different, but still very special."

Make some new traditions. Some people dealing with cancer have found new, deeply meaningful traditions. One woman's friend gave her a Christmas tree ornament and said, "Hang this on your tree this year and every year to come because you're going to beat this!" The woman told me, "I've hung that ornament on the tree for 22 Christmases now. It's a sign that I did prevail!"

Ask family and friends to help. Asking others to help can make a celebration more manageable. Maybe your Super Bowl party this year could be a potluck with everyone bringing a dish or two. Perhaps an aunt or uncle could lend a hand with your child's birthday party, or a good friend could prepare the Passover Seder meal. A survivor's brother said:

> "Cinco de Mayo is my sister's favorite holiday. She loves to cook and has a treasure trove of recipes handed down from our grandmother, who was born in Mexico. But after being diagnosed with cancer, she learned to let go somewhat and delegate. Her husband did the shopping and some of the food preparation. Her son-in-law, who's also a great cook, handled several of the more involved dishes, following her directions to the letter. She was able to spend much of the day resting in a comfy chair and enjoying the hustle and bustle around her."

Involving family and friends can lift a burden from your shoulders—and it can be a source of joy for them to help.

Pace yourself. Know your limits and give yourself plenty of time to rest. It's okay to decline some invitations or adjust certain activities. Cutting back a little on what you do conserves energy, reduces stress, and allows you to more fully enjoy the activities you choose to do. A survivor told me, "I went to my daughter's place for her Fourth of July party but didn't stay for the fireworks. Everybody seemed glad to see me there, even though I left early."

Be creative. One woman decided to attend her nephew's annual Halloween costume party, even though she was hesitant at first. Here's how she described it:

> "My treatment had caused me to lose my hair, so I found just the right wig and went dressed as Cleopatra. I didn't have a lot of energy, so I sat in a rocking chair for most of the party, looking regal and enjoying my nephew's family and friends. At one point, a few strapping young men decided to play the role of my servants, picking up my chair and carrying me around the room. I loved it!"

Accept whatever you're feeling. Holidays can be emotional times, so allow yourself to experience your feelings, whatever they may be. The message of chapter 8, "Don't Feel Bad about Feeling Bad," definitely applies during holidays—you don't have to pretend to be cheerful. In fact, the more someone feels compelled to appear happy, the less likely he or she is to actually feel happy. So if holidays are getting you down, don't get down on yourself. Accept and express your real feelings. With less pressure to feel good, you might actually feel a little better.

Stay open to the possibility that you could have a good time. Some people have told me that others' holiday cheer rubbed off on them. I've also heard from those who said they had just wanted to stay home and draw their shades until a holiday was over, but when they decided to go out to a party or celebration anyway, they had a good time. Don't push yourself beyond your physical or emotional limits, but if you think something might help you feel a little better, go for it. You may be surprised by how much you enjoy yourself.

One man shared his experience: "Easter was shortly after my surgery. I was still very weak, and I wasn't looking forward to going to my mom's house for the traditional family gathering. But I did go—and I'm glad I did. It was a surprisingly good day. Having my family around me was very uplifting."

Make memories. People dealing with cancer may worry about being a burden; they may think they'll put a damper on the festivities and ruin everyone else's fun. But those I've talked with have said that the opposite was true. The memories were even more special, family members valued each other even more, and the holiday took on an even deeper meaning. One survivor told me, "Thanksgiving that year was less about food and much more about being together. We talked more, shared story after story, and did a lot of laughing and hugging. I wouldn't trade that memory for anything. It was really special, and we've talked about it a lot in the years since."

Whatever limitations cancer might create for your holidays and celebrations, just do what you can and don't worry about what you can't. Focus on what matters most to you. When you make the most of holidays, they can continue to be a source of joy and solace for you.

43

Have a
Good Laugh

*"My son and a group of his high school friends all
shaved their heads to show their support after my
diagnosis. I was so touched that I invited them all over
for pizza. While they were visiting, I let them each
model a couple of old wigs people had given me, and
we took pictures of them looking like long-haired rock
stars. We laughed so hard that night. I'll never forget
how that group of teenagers lifted my spirits and
made me feel so normal."*

Just as it's good to cry as much as you need to, it's also good to laugh as much as you like. Whenever you feel like laughing, embrace it and laugh away.

In chapter 32, "Laughter Enhances the Best Medicine," I wrote about laughing with your medical team, but of course laughing is great any time. Laughter can be therapeutic. It's an excellent way to release tension and express your feelings. After a good laugh, things can seem a little lighter and easier to handle.

Now, you may be wondering, *How can there be anything for me to laugh about at a time like this?* Every now and then, however, humor comes up in daily life—a well-timed joke, an odd situation, or an unusual comment comes out of nowhere and strikes you as funny. When those unexpected moments occur, it can be good to let yourself laugh.

But you don't have to laugh if you don't feel like it. Trying to force or fake laughter when you're simply not in the mood can make you feel worse. Just let laughter come naturally, and welcome it when it does.

One woman talked about the heavy, solemn mood in her family while she was undergoing chemotherapy. Then one day, her five-year-old grandson innocently asked whether he could bring Granny to kindergarten show-and-tell so he could show off her bald head. "Everyone was very quiet at first," she said, "until I began to laugh. Then we all laughed—hard. Boy, that felt good!"

Laughing together can help people dealing with cancer to weather the storm. It can create happy memories during a difficult time. It can turn awkward moments into funny ones. Laughter can celebrate instances of grace and draw people closer together.

Here are several stories people with cancer and their loved ones have shared with me about times when they had a good laugh.

Forgetting the Wig

"I was out clothes-shopping with my daughter. In the dressing room, I took off my wig to try on an outfit. My daughter said from outside, 'Mom, come out, I want to see how it looks on you.' I walked out to show her—forgetting to put my wig back on—and just then the sales clerk came around the corner. When I saw her, my hands immediately flew to the top of my head. Right away, my daughter started laughing, and then I did too. To this day it still brings a smile to my face."

The Glow in the Dark Club

"Several of us who were going through treatment together became good friends. Since our treatment included the use of a radioactive isotope, we'd joke about glowing in the dark. We even got T-shirts with a neon orange radioactive symbol and the words 'Glow in the Dark Club.'"

"Grandma's Hair Came Back!"

"My grandson, who was in preschool, came to our home to visit. He asked about my hair, which I'd lost during chemotherapy, and I said, 'Oh, it's okay, it'll come back before long.' During another visit a few days later, he wandered into my bedroom, and when he saw my wig on the dresser, he ran into the kitchen and excitedly told his mother, 'It came back! Grandma's hair came back!' I just couldn't stop laughing about that."

The Secret to a Great Golf Game

"Strangely enough, shortly after one of my brother's chemotherapy treatments, he played his best round of golf ever. When he and his friends got together for their next outing, he told them he was willing to share the secret of his great game with them—and then took out a chemotherapy sign-up sheet he'd put together. For some reason, he didn't have any takers, but they all got a laugh out of it."

Trying a New Hairstyle

"When my hair started falling out, I decided to get it over with all at once—so I went to my hairdresser and said, 'Buzz it all off.' Then, just before she got started, I had a fun idea and told her, 'Before you shave it, I want a mohawk.' So she shaved the sides, dyed the rest purple, and got it sticking straight up. We took lots of pictures with me posing like a punk rocker with my purple mohawk. We had a great time, and I laughed so much I had to wipe away the tears."

There's nothing wrong with having a good laugh while you're dealing with cancer—or even laughing at the cancer itself. Laughing doesn't mean you're dismissing the seriousness of cancer. When something's funny, people laugh. Why let cancer take that away from you?

Laughter might not always come easily, but when it does, it can relieve tension and make your life a little bit better. So when the opportunity comes up to have a good laugh, go for it!

44

Forgive Others

"People who haven't had cancer might not know how to respond to those of us who do. Sometimes they say and do things that hurt me, even though they don't mean to. It's not always easy, but I'm learning to forgive them and just let it go."

Forgiveness is a powerful act. It benefits both the person doing the forgiving and the person being forgiven. When you have cancer (or even when you don't), forgiving others can do a world of good.

Forgiveness Is Choosing to Let Go

Forgiveness is a choice. When you forgive someone, you *choose* to let go of the bitterness or resentment you may feel, along with any intention to retaliate. It's a one-way action—something you do that requires nothing of the other person.

One man told me, "I finally said to myself, *I'm done letting this bother me. I'm simply not going to carry this grudge any longer.* Cancer was a heavy enough burden; carrying a sack of resentment on my back along with it just left me more exhausted. So it only made sense to set the sack down and stay focused on dealing with the cancer."

Clearing Up Some Misconceptions about Forgiveness

Here are some common misconceptions about forgiveness, along with the corresponding facts.

Misconception: In order to forgive, you have to forget what the other person did.

Fact: Forgiving does not require forgetting. The hurt might stay with you for a while—you are simply choosing not to dwell on it anymore.

Misconception: When you forgive someone, you are giving that person permission to continue to hurt you.

Fact: Forgiveness does not mean allowing others to walk all over you. By forgiving, you aren't saying it was okay for the other person to do what he or she did. You can forgive while still setting boundaries and making it clear that certain behaviors are unacceptable to you.

Misconception: Forgiving someone will cause him or her to stop behaving in hurtful ways.

Fact: Your forgiveness might not change a thing about the other person. The other person may or may not behave better in the future. That's not the point of forgiveness. It's about changing your life for the better, not about trying to change someone else's behavior.

Misconception: The other person needs to say, "I'm sorry," before you forgive him or her.

Fact: You don't have to wait for an apology in order to forgive. It's possible that the person isn't going to apologize or doesn't even realize that he or she did something hurtful. Regardless of whether the person has said, "I'm sorry," you can forgive him or her.

Misconception: It isn't real forgiveness unless you tell the other person that he or she is forgiven.

Fact: Forgiveness doesn't mean you have to tell the other person, "I forgive you." In some instances, you might tell the person you forgive him or her, but you can also forgive someone internally and privately.

Misconception: You can't forgive someone unless you also settle your differences with him or her.

Fact: You can forgive without trying to resolve a disagreement or reconcile a relationship. The most important part of forgiveness is personal—your decision to let go of your resentment. Whether you also attempt to resolve the issue or restore the relationship is a different matter.

Benefits of Forgiving

Forgiveness can bring significant benefits.

Forgiveness can cut off the negative power another person is wielding in your life. When you let go of resentment, you free yourself from that hurtful influence.

Forgiveness can lighten your load. Forgiving someone allows you to set down excess emotional baggage so you can move forward with more ease and grace. As one person with cancer put it, "Forgiving released me from the anger and bitterness that weighed down my heart."

Forgiveness can be a first step toward restoring a relationship. I've heard from people who were able to rebuild loving relationships with estranged friends and family members once they chose to forgive.

Forgiveness lets you take control of your emotions—instead of allowing them to control you. It can lead to greater peace of mind and free up energy that you can invest in taking care of yourself.

Overcoming Challenges to Forgiveness

Forgiving isn't always easy to do; it can involve overcoming some challenges. Here are a few suggestions for how to handle those challenges.

Be patient with yourself. Don't worry if forgiving takes longer than you thought it would. It's not always easy to forgive others when they've wronged you and caused you pain. It may take some time before you're able to forgive. Give yourself the time you need—you don't have to push yourself to forgive before you're ready.

Try to understand the other person. One way someone can take a step toward forgiveness is by trying to understand what was going on inside the other person. For instance, was he or she possibly frightened and at a loss for words in the presence of someone dealing with cancer? In a desperate attempt to say something kind, did he or she unintentionally say something hurtful instead? Asking questions like these can make it easier to forgive.

One person told me, "What often helps me to let go of hurtful things people say or do is to consider the circumstances. Some are well-meaning folks who just don't know how to relate to someone with cancer. Others speak without thinking. And others want to 'bless' me with everything they know. I just try to understand and move on."

Talk with someone about spiritual challenges with forgiveness. For many people, the act of forgiveness is closely tied to their faith. If this is true for you, it may be helpful to find someone you can talk to about any spiritual struggles you are having with forgiveness (see chapter 72, "Seek Out Spiritual Community").

Forgive them for your sake, not theirs. Sometimes people do things that are so mean or hurtful that, no matter how much you try, you just can't understand why. They may not even acknowledge having hurt you, and they might not seem to care how what they did has affected you. Such circumstances can make it more difficult to let go and forgive.

In these situations, you might choose to forgive because it's the most healing thing you can do for yourself. You also might choose to forgive someone who seems totally undeserving because you know how much you've been forgiven. You're the one who chooses your reasons to forgive.

Forgiving Brings Freedom

I certainly can't say you have to forgive others. I don't know the wrongs you've experienced or the pain in your heart. But I can tell you this: Forgiving is good for you. It can reduce your stress and increase your energy. It can free you from painful memories, empower you to move forward in life, and make you feel better about yourself and those around you. It can heal broken hearts and restore damaged relationships. As difficult as forgiving can be, it is well worth doing when you're able.

A cancer survivor once told me, "I have a choice: I can let something eat at me, or I can forgive, let it go, and move on with my life." When you forgive, you open yourself to living as fully, freely, and lovingly as you can.

45

Forgive Yourself

"I've finally stopped beating myself up for waiting so long to have a colonoscopy. For a while, I was really angry at myself, but what good does that do? I need to focus my energy on getting better."

If forgiving others is difficult at times, forgiving ourselves can be even harder. But forgiving yourself can be just as beneficial—or even more so.

Just as forgiving others means letting go of bitterness or resentment toward another person, self-forgiveness means letting go of such feelings toward yourself. One man told me, "When I was first diagnosed, I was really hard on myself. I'd look in the mirror and blame myself for just about everything. Then I realized that I was wasting a lot of time and energy. I needed to stop going after the man in the mirror and fight the cancer instead."

We All Need Self-Forgiveness at Times

Just about everyone feels regret or self-blame at one time or another, and cancer can amplify such feelings. We may feel bad about something we know is our fault—maybe we said or did something and later wished we hadn't, or maybe we could have helped someone but didn't. All of us have something to forgive ourselves for. As one person with cancer said, "Of course I had to forgive myself. My anger, impatience, frustration, or fear boiled over at times. Then I'd realize how I'd acted and think, *Yikes! I can't believe I did that.*"

Other times we may dwell on something that really isn't our fault; we didn't actually do anything wrong, but we feel bad anyway. It can help to realize we have nothing to forgive ourselves for in those instances. That realization can free us to let go of any remorse we feel.

Clearing Up Some Misconceptions about Forgiving Ourselves

It's important to clear up some misconceptions that could prevent us from forgiving ourselves.

Misconception: If I forgive myself, it means I'm denying that I did anything wrong.

Fact: Forgiving myself begins with recognizing that I did something I wish I hadn't—or that I didn't do something I wish I had—and feeling sorry about it.

Misconception: If I forgive myself for a mistake, it means I don't take my mistake seriously.

Fact: Forgiving myself isn't a way to dismiss mistakes—to say that particular words or actions don't really matter. Rather, it includes acknowledging that my behavior may have hurt myself or others.

Misconception: Forgiving myself gives me permission to repeat potentially harmful behaviors.

Fact: Part of forgiving myself is owning up to what I've done wrong, making amends whenever possible, avoiding behaviors that might hurt myself or others, and intending to live as responsibly as I can in the future.

Misconception: I can forgive myself only if I'm sure I'll never make the same mistake again.

Fact: Forgiving myself includes remaining aware that I'm human—I'm not perfect and never will be. If I refuse to forgive myself because I'm afraid I might fall short again, I'm setting too high a standard. Nobody can live without mistakes and missteps. In spite of my best intentions, I may repeat the same misdeed and need to forgive myself again.

Benefits of Forgiving Yourself

Forgiving yourself can have significant benefits.

Forgiving yourself can bring emotional freedom. Punishing yourself for past mistakes won't change anything. When you choose to forgive yourself, it releases you from the burden of self-criticism and anger weighing you down.

Forgiving yourself can free up energy for dealing with cancer. Self-reproach saps your energy; it can exhaust you. Forgiving yourself liberates you to focus your strength on fighting the cancer instead. One person with cancer said, "It took me a while, but I was able to let my self-blame go. That freed up a lot of energy that I could spend on other things—like getting better."

Forgiving yourself can help build relationships. Constant self-criticism can get in the way of relationships with people you love; it puts up barriers to constructive relating and communicating. When you forgive yourself, you can remove those barriers and build relationships that bring comfort and strength to you and your loved ones.

Suggestions to Help with Forgiving Yourself

If you're struggling with feelings of regret or anger at yourself, these suggestions may help you forgive yourself.

View yourself as a compassionate outside observer would. If someone you love were struggling with painful feelings of guilt in the midst of coping with cancer, you'd probably have tremendous compassion for him or her. Try to have that kind of compassion for yourself.

Talk with someone you can trust. You might share your difficult feelings with a close friend, a family member, a kindred spirit, members of a support group, or a professional counselor. Many times, just talking about such feelings is a good way to let them go.

Talk about spiritual matters. As the previous chapter mentioned, it may help to talk to someone about the spiritual aspects of forgiveness (see chapter 72, "Seek Out Spiritual Community").

Turn your "if onlys" into "next times." Instead of beating yourself up for what you did or didn't do in the past, decide what you intend to do differently in the future. Invest your energy in "next times" rather than "if onlys." Put self-judgment behind you, and focus on saying and doing things differently from now on. One survivor put it this way: "Wishing for a different past is a waste of energy. I can't change what I've already done. I can only change what I do from now on."

Be patient and persistent with yourself. Sometimes forgiving yourself for something just once isn't enough—you might still find yourself dwelling on it from time to time. You may need to forgive yourself for the same thing again and again before you finally move beyond those feelings.

Ask for forgiveness. If you've said or done something that has hurt someone else, apologizing and asking that person for forgiveness can be healing. No matter how the person responds, your apology can pave the way for you to forgive yourself.

Forgiving yourself, like forgiving anyone else, can take time. You might need to work at it for a while. But the relief, freedom, and self-acceptance you'll feel are worth it. One person told me, "In addition to my tumor, I discovered something else was hurting me—self-blaming. Its symptoms were: 'I could have,' 'I would have,' 'I should have,' 'What if,' 'If only,' 'Why didn't I,' and 'What might have been.' The only treatment for it was to forgive myself."

46

Accept Help

"Because of the long recovery after surgery and the effects of chemotherapy, I couldn't pull my own weight like I used to. I was always the person who took care of everyone else. Now, I needed care, and I had to learn to let people give me a helping hand."

You don't have to stand alone against cancer. There are family, friends, colleagues, neighbors—and perhaps even others you don't know yet—who may express their willingness to provide the kinds of help and support you need.

I encourage you to accept their offers and allow them to help you.

This can be trickier than it sounds, because we often want to be as independent as possible. We may have trouble accepting help, even when we're dealing with cancer. We may tell ourselves and others, "I'm okay. I can handle this." One survivor told me, "At first, I was too embarrassed to let others help me. Not being able to cope on my own just didn't seem right."

Also, some people get so used to helping others that they find it difficult to turn the tables and allow others to help them. A man with cancer said, "It's always been much easier for me to do things for others than to let them do things for me. But my family overruled my objections and stepped in to help, and I was glad they did."

Your Own Personal Natural Disaster

Think of it this way. Every time a natural disaster hits, like a tornado or an earthquake, we see story after story about people showing up and helping out. We admire those who pitch in, and we're glad to see people receiving the support and assistance they need when their lives have been turned upside down.

You've experienced your own personal tornado or earthquake, so when people offer you their help, by all means accept it if it truly meets your needs. With all the changes and challenges that cancer brings, nobody should have to face it alone.

Accepting Help Is a Sign of Strength

It's all right to accept help as you need it. You're not a superhero; you don't need to manage everything on your own. Leaning on others as necessary is nothing to be ashamed of. We're all human, and we all have limits. Recognizing your limits and saying when you need help shows strength, not weakness.

Sometimes you may need someone to assist with chores and responsibilities, such as preparing meals, doing yard work, housecleaning, running errands, transporting children, or driving you or your loved one to appointments. Other times, you may just want someone to be there to provide company or take your mind off things. One person shared, "Sometimes all I needed was for someone to come over and watch TV with me, or sit with me on the porch, or take me out to look at the autumn leaves." Whatever kind of help you need, feel free to ask for it and receive it.

Accepting Help Can Give Caregivers a Chance to Rest

Accepting help can provide primary caregivers a much-needed opportunity to recharge as well. One man described his experience:

> "I'm a pretty private person, and I was reluctant to receive help from others. But I trusted my wife, and I felt okay about her helping me. Then a friend offered to drive me to an appointment, and I said that my wife could take care of it. He said, 'She's taking care of a lot already. Let me help out with this one.' That made me realize that when I accepted help for me, I was also accepting help for my wife. I decided to get past my reluctance and receive help from others for both of our sakes."

Accepting Help Is a Gift to Your Helpers

When you accept help, you're also offering a gift to those who want to help you. There are people who truly want to give you assistance and support. It brings them joy and satisfaction to know that they're able to make your life a little easier.

One man told me, "I've always been quick to help others, and I know how good it feels to lend a hand. So when I was the one in need, I realized that if I didn't accept other people's offers, I was denying them the same satisfaction. When one person helps another, both are blessed."

A woman said, "I turned down people's offers of help until I got really weak during chemo. Letting them support me in various ways made my life easier, but I also saw how good it made them feel. They'd been feeling helpless in the face of my illness, and having the chance to do something for me boosted their morale. Now I wish I'd started saying yes much sooner!"

Of course, people will be most helpful when they know *how* to help. So it's to your advantage—and theirs too—when you offer specific suggestions about the kinds of assistance you need most (see chapter 58, "Tell Others What You Need").

It's good to accept offers of help that come your way. People who care about you are eager to assist you during this challenging time. By welcoming their help, you make it easier for yourself and your loved ones, and you also give them a gift in return: the joy of helping you.

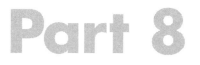

Part 8

Relating to Immediate Family

47

Cancer Upsets
the Family Dynamic

*"Dad's cancer diagnosis knocked our entire
family for a loop. It brought all sorts of
new challenges, which led to emotions and
reactions we had never witnessed before.
It was raw, uncharted territory for us."*

Cancer affects the whole family. Only one person might have the disease, but the entire family can be turned upside down by it. One survivor reflected:

"Cancer wears and tears on family members, both physically and emotionally. It puts them through so many changes so quickly, and they feel helpless to stop it. They want you to feel better, and they try so hard to think of things that can help you. They hurt inside when they see you suffering or if they think you're in pain. It's hard for them to watch you undergo those treatments and surgeries. Their lives are put on hold while you go through all this."

This chapter focuses on some of the stressful situations your family might experience. Just being aware of these challenges is a start. Then, the next few chapters offer strategies for working through them as a family.

Juggling Roles and Responsibilities

It's possible that family members will have to shift roles and take on new responsibilities. The primary income provider might need to add cooking, cleaning, grocery shopping, and childcare to his or her list of responsibilities. A spouse who has stayed home to raise children may need to find employment. Responsibility for managing finances may fall to a family member who has never had to deal with such issues before. A teenager might have to take on more tasks around the house. A younger child, in need of care and reassurance, may instead feel the need to take care of others.

A woman described the changes that occurred when she was a child and her older sister was being treated for cancer:

> "Mom was busy driving my sister back and forth to the hospital. Dad was busy trying to cook and maintain the house, as well as work. I was little, but I pitched in every way I could. Our family life completely changed. We were just trying to get through each day."

All these new roles, expectations, and challenges can disrupt routines and knock the family out of balance. Family members may struggle to handle new responsibilities on top of all they currently do, leaving them feeling overwhelmed and exhausted.

A man described how complicated life became when family roles had to change after his diagnosis:

> "When it came to dealing with hard issues in our family, I had always been the strong and positive one, so I didn't think I could tell them that I was coming apart at the seams. But one day, halfway through my treatments, I realized that I just couldn't take care of everyone like that anymore, and I broke down.

> "After that, I told my family that I needed them to be the strong ones now and take care of me. We were scared at first, but big role changes took place. They learned to care for me, and I learned how to tell them what I needed and let them help. We all made it through the changes together and even grew because of them."

Financial Challenges

In many families, cancer also creates financial challenges. It may not be possible to work while going through treatment, and the family may lose a source of income. Plus, cancer treatment can involve some major expenses, which can lead to sacrifices in the family budget, as well as mounting debt. Complicated bills and insurance forms take time to sift through, which can cause further stress.

Distance Challenges

Cancer can be even more challenging when family members live a long distance from one another. Those who live far away may feel bad because they aren't there to support their loved one in person. One family member told me:

> "When I got the call from Mom, I didn't know what to say or do. I wished more than anything that I could have been there with her right then. It's hard to give someone a hug when you're living on the other side of the country."

A woman recounted:

> "My two grown daughters lived far away with their husbands and children. My younger daughter took time off from work to be with me for my first surgery, and my older daughter did the same for my second surgery. I remember crying and telling them, 'I never wanted to be a burden to anyone,' but they assured me that they really wanted to help."

Family Conflict

When cancer enters the picture, it can bring conflict. A survivor told me, "People under a lot of stress sometimes say hurtful things to those they love and care for, even when they need each other the most." A hospital chaplain said, "Cancer can bring old wounds and conflicts to the surface. People can react badly when they're scared."

Different ways of coping can cause friction between family members. The mother of a child with cancer told me, "One parent can be in denial while the other desperately needs to talk and take action. Differences like that can lead to conflict."

Plans for the Future

Cancer can throw a family's plans for the future into question. Plans for the immediate future—like vacations, family reunions, or college—may need to be changed. Letting go of activities that everyone was looking forward to can be very disappointing.

One survivor described her experience: "We had to postpone many of our future plans and focus on living in the now. We didn't think so much about what we were going to do in a month or in a year. It took all we had just to deal with today and tomorrow."

Challenges for Those Who Are Single

People who are single or living alone may face additional family-related challenges after a cancer diagnosis. They may at times need help from family, or they may end up moving in with a family member in order to get needed support. It can be difficult to fend for yourself when you're alone, but reaching out to others for help can bring an unwelcome sense of dependency, even when it's necessary.

One woman said:

> "Because I'm a single parent, I had to hold on to a lot of the roles I had before the cancer, and it wore me out. My sister from out of state was able to come for a while after my surgery and help take care of the boys. It was a real godsend, but I felt guilty about pulling her away from her family for that time, even though she said she was glad to do this for me."

Changes to Children's Routines

When a family member has cancer, it often changes routines for everyone in the family, and children may have an especially difficult time adapting. A survivor said, "Parents with cancer may not be able to attend their children's sporting events or music recitals. If there's someone who helps care for the children, that person may not do everything the same way the parents do. Children can become upset or confused by the changes to their comfortable routine and may not know how to express those feelings."

Hunger for Normalcy

All the changes and stresses caused by cancer can leave family members yearning for how things used to be. One person described family life with cancer this way:

> "There's no way to maintain normalcy. Sometimes everything seems to revolve around the cancer and the patient. The stress and the fear are there when you go to bed, and they're still there when you wake up. After a few weeks of doctor visits and telling everyone the news, all you crave is normalcy, but it's nowhere to be found. Your loved one with cancer needs normalcy too and wants it more than anything. The tension created by this need and the inability to meet it can be overwhelming at times."

These Changes Aren't Anyone's Fault

When cancer hits, what was once normal and routine no longer is. The family faces changes and challenges, as well as the stress that comes with them. As you encounter these challenges, it's vital to remember that *none of this is your fault.* You didn't upset the family dynamic—the cancer did.

The other chapters in this section provide ideas for how families can move through these challenges together.

48

Everyone
Reacts Differently

"I was unprepared for the variety of emotions that affected people in my family. I thought we'd all respond in pretty much the same way, but we didn't. Each member of my family had to find his or her own way of coping with the cancer."

No two people react the same way to cancer. This is true for people with cancer—and it's just as true for their family members.

Each family member will have different feelings and ways of responding to the diagnosis and coping with the day-to-day realities of cancer. Here's how one woman described it:

> "My family has dealt with cancer several times, and I can tell you from personal experience that people respond in a lot of different ways. Some pull away; others draw closer. Some behave irresponsibly; others get more dependable. Some people become more caring and loving, others less so. How people react can cover the whole waterfront. That's just how people are. I've learned that cancer can bring out the best—and the worst—in us."

I won't try to list all the ways family members might react to cancer, but here are examples that people have shared with me. Perhaps some will be similar to your own experience.

> "My son was in a state of disbelief for months; he didn't know what to say, so he said very little. My daughter spent every spare moment on the internet, digging up any possible treatments and bits of advice she could. My husband mostly helped in practical ways—he didn't talk

a lot about my cancer because he didn't want to add to my burden. I know, though, that he sometimes talked with coworkers to let his worries out."

"When my grandpa got cancer, my brother became very angry and hard to get along with. When I tried to talk with him about it, he'd yell and walk out. He'd always been close to our grandpa, and he just didn't know how to deal with it."

"When I was diagnosed, my older daughter was 14, a freshman starting high school, and my younger daughter was 11. The older one was uncomfortable with visible reminders of my disease; she wanted me to look like my normal self as much as possible. But as soon as I'd get home, the younger one would say, 'Mom, take off that wig and get that sweat off your face.'"

"My dad tried to ignore the situation and act as if nothing was going on. He didn't avoid me; he just didn't talk about my cancer or how he felt about it. And if I brought it up, he'd change the subject as soon as he could. Ever since I was a child he's had a difficult time talking about feelings."

"My daughter was a doer; she wanted to bring me the paper, get me water, and do other things so I could rest. My son cheered me on, drawing me pictures and making me cards. My wife worked to keep everything organized and make sure we were all doing okay. We didn't do it perfectly, but we helped each other through a really tough time."

"My wife wanted to learn as much as she could about the disease. My first daughter, our oldest child, was concerned about every decision, a lot like her mom—should I do this or that? My older son asked no questions about the cancer; he was afraid to deal with the subject. My younger son often asked about me and about the prognosis and reports, but he quickly got on to other topics. My younger daughter always prayed for me and shared her prayers with me. All five of them loved me and cared about how I was doing, but each expressed it differently."

Members of your family may react like the people in any of these examples, or their responses may be something else entirely. I'm sharing these stories to make this point: Different people can have completely different reactions when faced with a crisis like cancer. As a clinical psychologist and a pastor, I've seen people react in a wide variety of ways to crises, from intense sobbing to stoic acceptance, from energetic support to stunned silence, and everything in between.

People are like that. In the face of cancer, everyone reacts differently, and you may not be able to predict how people will respond, even those closest to you. Recognizing this can make it easier to handle such a range of reactions.

49

Go Easy on
Each Other

*"While dealing with cancer, we sometimes got
irritable with each other and made a big deal
out of small problems. It just happened. The
only way we got through this was to work on
treating each other with gentleness, kindness,
patience, and understanding."*

As different family members react to the stress of cancer in their own
ways, it's beneficial for everyone to go easy on each other. Doing so can
help your family work together against the cancer.

Here are a couple of ways you can go easy on each other.

Cut Each Other Some Slack

When people are dealing with cancer, they won't always perform or relate
at their best. They may not take care of household responsibilities as well
as before. They may not be as considerate as you've come to expect. One
woman who had cancer told me, "Life was so discombobulated; it seemed
like 'please' and 'thank you' went out the window."

You and your family may do better if all of you relax your expectations
a bit. If you're used to your home being neat and orderly, you may choose
to accept some disarray during this time. If certain family members seem
preoccupied with their own needs and less aware of what others require, it
can help to remember the pressure you're all under and not expect everyone
to be on his or her best behavior right now.

One person said:

"For a while after my diagnosis, my teenage stepdaughter barely said a word to us and never even mentioned my cancer. My husband was frustrated by what seemed like her lack of interest in my condition. I told him to be patient—that she cared but just needed time to sort things out. Then one day she came to me and asked, 'Can we talk? I'm really scared.' After that heart-to-heart conversation, she was much more like herself."

Cancer puts everyone in the family under a lot of stress. In such a situation, it's not always easy to cut each other some slack, but doing so is a great way to care for one another during a very difficult time.

Families can benefit from talking about expectations and agreeing to relax them when possible. A survivor said:

"As a family of six, we had a weekly list of chores for each person. Normally the tasks were manageable, but life with cancer was not normal. So we sat down and decided which chores could be done less frequently and which could be given to people who had offered to help us. That relieved a lot of pressure for everyone."

Give Each Other the Benefit of the Doubt

If someone says or does something that seems hurtful, it can be easy to jump to the conclusion that he or she is doing it on purpose, which can make you feel even worse. Instead, it's much easier on everyone when family members give each other the benefit of the doubt—when they think the best about one another rather than assuming that others' words and actions are intended to hurt.

The son of a woman with cancer shared this story:

"I remember one time when my sister and I were in the kitchen, preparing a meal for the family because Mom wasn't able to. We got into an argument over something minor, and our tempers really flared up for a minute or two. I started blaming her, like I did when we were kids. But then I realized, *It's no one's fault. We're both just afraid for Mom. That's all—it's nothing personal.* That realization helped me let go of my anger, apologize for my part, and talk it out with her. Whenever we got short-tempered after that, I tried to keep that in mind: *It's not personal; we're just afraid.*"

One survivor recounted her experience:

"I had to learn that when I heard something that may have been insensitive, it was almost always someone speaking out of his or her own pain, confusion, and fear, not someone trying to hurt me. It helped to stop and remember that before I responded."

A woman told me:

"We had several relatives who stopped calling and visiting when they learned of the diagnosis. It hurt at first, but we figured they were probably shocked and upset and didn't know what to say or do, so we left the door open to get back together when they were ready."

Certainly, at times you may need to hold others accountable for their actions. If someone is causing harm to you or others, it's important to address that, letting the person know kindly but firmly that his or her behavior is hurtful and needs to change. But in most instances, simply going easy on each other helps everyone out.

One cancer survivor put it this way: "Relax. Don't get bent out of shape. When a family member has cancer, getting all worked up over little things doesn't do any good. If someone isn't communicating or acting perfectly, you might be able to take a deep breath and roll with it." So, as you are able, try to go easy on each other.

50

Share What You're Feeling

"I was raised in a 'we-don't-talk-about-our-emotions'
family, so when my husband would ask me, 'How are you
feeling?' I would talk about things like fatigue or nausea.
Once I realized what he was really asking, I discovered
how much more I had to tell him. Talking about my
frustrations, worries, and joys drew us closer together
and helped me feel better."

When you're dealing with cancer, there may be times when you just need to talk—to share what you're feeling.

A survivor told me, "There were days when my husband would come home from work, and I'd say, 'I need to talk.' I'd tell him whether it had been a hard day or a better day and talk about all the ups and downs, and he would listen. Getting all that out would help me feel better afterwards."

When you think it would help to share your thoughts and feelings with a family member, go ahead and do so. It can be a great source of relief as well as a powerful way to strengthen relationships.

Examples of People Sharing Feelings with Their Families

Here are some situations where people found it helpful to share their feelings with others in the family:

"My sister came for a visit from out of state. One of the first things she did was to sit me down, take my hand, and say, 'Okay, go ahead and unload.' I poured out all my frustrations over trying to balance my job, children, housework, and everything else, all while taking care of my husband who had cancer. I was worn out, and I really needed to tell someone about it."

"I was living with my parents when I was diagnosed, and I remember telling them how bad I felt about the disruption my cancer was going to cause for the entire family. I shared my worries about the pressure I'd be putting on them, along with everything else that was coming our way. They assured me they could handle it, and I was glad I spoke up."

"I came by the hospital to visit my dad after his surgery. After chatting about nothing in particular for a while, he just looked at me and said, 'You know I love you, don't you?' And I said, 'Yes, Daddy, I do.' He'd never been the kind of person to talk about his feelings, but we've grown so much closer since that day."

"Being diagnosed with cancer left me with all these emotions I wasn't ready for. I was heartbroken for my wife and our children—how would this affect them? I was worried about all the unknowns ahead of me, about what *would* happen and what *could* happen. So I called my mom and talked about what was on my mind. It was good to get all that out."

The Power of Sharing

There is power in honestly sharing your feelings, especially difficult feelings. Here's what a number of people have told me about the ways sharing their feelings with a family member helped them.

Sharing Can Calm Turbulent Feelings

Unexpressed feelings can churn inside and cause a lot of discomfort, but sharing can help calm those feelings and bring them under control.

"About a week after my diagnosis, I had my first real chance to share what had built up inside. I visited my sister and just let out my fears and uncertainties about my family's future. She listened the whole time, and a sense of calm came over me. I look back now, and I believe that she was a gift from God for me that day."

$\sim$

"My brother and I had always had a good relationship. We called each other often, and we went fishing together once a year. But the year he was fighting cancer, we talked at least once a week. I shared feelings with him that I couldn't tell anyone else, and I know he did the same with me. And, of course, we told fishing stories. After it was all behind him, he told me, 'I always knew that you were there for me and that I could tell you anything. It gave me such relief.'"

Sharing Can Lighten the Load

When the stress of dealing with a cancer diagnosis weighs you down, sharing what you're experiencing can lighten the load.

"I remember one day when things got too heavy for me to deal with on my own. I called my mom and said, 'I need you,' and she came right over. When she got there, I spent about an hour letting it all out. Then I just lay there with my head in her lap—the only time I've done that in my adult life. That was a precious moment of relief for me. My mom was there to care for me; I wasn't facing this cancer all alone."

Sharing Can Relieve Pressure

The stress brought about by cancer can build up inside like steam in a pressure cooker. Sharing is like a vent pipe that releases the distress.

"After my diagnosis, I closed off my emotions and didn't communicate about them at all. I didn't voice my fears or talk about my cancer. I just held it all in and tried to live in a bubble, above it all. But one day that bubble burst. My raw emotions spilled out—I talked and talked for a long time while my son and daughter-in-law listened. I found that talking about my scariest feelings helped me get them out of my system and actually made life easier."

$\sim$

"As his treatments wore on, my brother-in-law opened up one day about the worries that were keeping him awake at night. Afterward, he took a deep breath and said, 'I'm glad we talked about this.' I could hear the relief in his voice and see it on his face."

Sharing Can Encourage Others to Share

Sharing often invites more sharing. When one person breaks the ice and talks about what he or she is feeling, it can clear the path for others to do so as well.

> "My family doesn't do feelings well, so our initial phone calls were mostly about physical stuff like my test results, treatments, and side effects. If I got emotional at all, there'd be an awkward pause, and then they'd try to change the subject. But over time, as I talked about my feelings, my brothers and sisters began to open up too. We'd talk about how much we cared for each other or what they were experiencing. If it was a bad day, they'd cry with me. If it was a good day, they'd be excited with me."

> "My wife has a tendency to hold things in—she almost never cries when anyone else is around. After her diagnosis, she showed very little emotion at first, but I could tell how troubled she was. One afternoon, while she was lying on the bed, I curled up next to her and held her. After a few minutes, I said, 'I'm scared.' When I said that, she started crying and opened up about her feelings, about all the fears and unknowns. She told me later that she really felt better getting that off her shoulders, and since then she's talked more openly to me about what's bothering her."

Sharing Can Strengthen Relationships

Cancer can strain relationships between family members. Sharing feelings is a way of moving past relational barriers and nurturing the bonds with the people who mean so much to you.

> "If I hadn't been talking to my wife through the whole thing, all my frustration and anger would have just stayed inside, and I would have become a hard person to get along with. Being able to tell her about all this stuff kept our relationship on an even keel while everything else seemed to be spiraling out of control."

"A few years ago, my oldest daughter called and said she had found some lumps in her breast and had just received a cancer diagnosis. Our relationship had always been a bit strained, but her need took priority. The first thing we did was to say straight out that we loved each other. From that moment on, as we've shared from our hearts, our relationship has slowly but surely grown deeper."

"After my dad's initial surgery, he felt a real need to open up to us. He said he'd always loved us, but he had trouble expressing it. He did all he could to provide for us, but he didn't always connect emotionally. Now, though, he said, 'I want to do more than just provide—I want to love.' Since then he's been much more willing to talk about his love for us, his struggles, and his fears. We've grown so much closer and loved so much deeper because of that."

Sharing Is *Not* a Pity Party

One time, I was talking with a friend who was struggling through a number of challenges, including cancer. I could tell he was hurting, so I listened as he filled me in on everything that was going on. After a while, he stopped in mid-sentence and said, "I'm sorry about going on and on like this. I didn't mean to have a pity party."

I didn't think he was whining or seeking pity at all. He was simply sharing his story and telling me about his feelings in a natural and appropriate way, and I told him so.

There is nothing wrong with letting out your emotional pain when you're hurting—with cancer or with anything else. Sharing your feelings in an honest and direct manner is perfectly healthy. It's not a pity party.

Sharing Brings Relief and Growth

Of course, as healthy as it can be, sharing your feelings with family members may not be easy. I've heard from people who've found it challenging to share. It may take time for you and your family to become comfortable talking about the emotions stirred up by cancer.

But it's well worth the effort to experience the power of sharing, to know the relief and relational growth it can bring to you and your family. In the next three chapters, I'll cover some ways family members can help each other share a little more easily.

51

Ask Others
How They're Doing

"When my sister had breast cancer, I'd regularly ask her how she was doing, and she'd share a lot. Then one day I asked her husband how he was feeling about all that was happening. He said, 'You're probably the first person who's asked me that.' After we talked, he told me that just having the chance to share his feelings gave him renewed strength."

Sharing feelings certainly brings a lot of benefits to a person with cancer and the rest of the family. For many people, though, sharing doesn't happen easily. They may be uncomfortable talking about their feelings, or they may not know that it's all right to share. It's often necessary for someone to jumpstart the sharing process so that others are more comfortable opening up and saying what's on their minds.

The best way to get sharing started is simply to ask other family members how they're doing and what they're feeling.

A cancer survivor told me, "I was reluctant to talk about my feelings, but that changed when my sister-in-law asked me to share. She said, 'I'm having trouble dealing with this, but I can't imagine how hard it is on you. I'd like to know how you're doing right now.'"

A man shared with me, "When my wife was in the midst of her cancer treatments, my teenage son would ask me, 'How are you doing, Dad—really?' His desire for honesty was both challenging and refreshing. The conversations we had brought us closer together."

Asking Lets People Know It's All Right to Share

When you ask people how they're doing, you're letting them know that it's all right for them to share. This is important because sometimes people don't think they have permission to talk honestly about what they're going through. Other times, they may hold back their feelings for fear of saddening or troubling their loved ones.

One woman said, "I didn't want to talk to my siblings about what a hard time I was having with Mom's cancer. I was afraid I wouldn't be able to handle my own feelings, and I thought letting them out would upset everyone else even more. But then my older sister said, 'It's okay. Just tell me about it.' Her asking opened the floodgates. I was so glad she brought it up."

A friend told me, "One day I got a text message from my brother saying, 'Bad day. I hate cancer.' I thought about texting him right back, but it sounded like he really needed to talk, so I called and said, 'What's happening?' He did some much-needed venting—I was glad I called."

How to Ask Family Members How They're Doing

Here are some suggestions for how you might ask family members about their feelings.

Ask Simply

Often, the best questions for getting at feelings are simple ones, like:

- "How are you doing today?"
- "I'd really like to know how you're feeling."
- "What's this like for you right now?"
- "What's on your mind today?"

Be ready with follow-up questions or statements such as "Tell me more," or "How are you doing with all this?"

Ask Directly

Be direct when you ask a family member how he or she is doing. That lets the other person know that you truly want to hear what's going on.

> "In the hard days after my diagnosis, my mother was candid and direct. She'd say, 'Tell me how you're doing. I'm your mom. You can talk to me just like you did when you would come home from a tough day at school.' It really helped me to tell her about all the questions and fears I had."

"At one point during my husband's treatment, I could tell he was holding it all in, trying to be strong for me. So I said to him, 'Honey, for 20 years you've always been there for me—and I appreciate that. But this time, I need to be there for you. Tell me what you're feeling. Tell me what you're thinking. Let me be there for you.'"

⁓

"Since I was the one who visited Dad most frequently to help him out, family members would call me for updates. One day my brother called and asked, 'How are you doing?' I started to talk about Dad, but he interrupted and said, 'Sis, I asked about you. You're right there, taking care of Dad. That must be really hard. How are *you* doing?' I got shaky and told him, 'I'm sad and I'm scared.'"

Ask Attentively

Pay attention to signals like tone of voice, body language, and general behavior, and then ask about what you notice.

"My daughter was very observant; she could tell by my voice whether I was feeling well. Sometimes when I was talking with her, she'd say, 'Mom, you don't sound like you feel good.' That helped me tell her what was going on inside."

⁓

"My husband could always sense my moods. If I wasn't saying anything, he knew something was wrong. So he'd say, 'You're not very talkative today. What's going on?' And then we'd talk it out."

Ask Again, as Needed

Sometimes a family member may be reluctant to share and may not give a full response the first time you ask. It's good to ask again as needed and encourage the person to say what's on his or her mind.

"One day my mother was lying in bed, exhausted from chemotherapy. As I sat next to her in a rocking chair, she made a fist and began to pound on the mattress. I put my hand on her shoulder and said, 'You seem angry. Want to talk about it?' She replied, 'I'm not angry.' So I said, 'Then why are you beating the snot out of your bed?' She burst into tears and cried out, 'I just don't understand. What did I do to deserve this? This isn't fair.'"

"Once when I asked our teenage son how he was doing, he looked at the floor and said in a soft voice, 'Oh, fine, I guess.' I put my hand on his shoulder and said, 'Fine?' He looked up at me and just laid it out. We had a great conversation, and since then we've had many more like it."

"My sister and I are very close. One time during my daughter's treatments, my sister asked me, 'How are you?' I said, 'I'm doing okay—tired but okay.' She waited a moment, looking at me caringly, and said, 'Go on, finish that thought. Tell me more about what you mean by 'tired but okay.'"

Ask in the Right Setting

Sometimes people are more responsive with their sharing when the setting is right. Often that's a quiet place or a private moment.

"When I felt strong enough, my husband and I would walk the dogs together. After a while of just walking, he'd say, 'So what are you thinking?' I always felt free to tell him everything in the solitude of those walks."

"When our little brother had cancer many years ago, my sister and I sometimes needed to get away from grownups and have some time to ourselves. So we'd get on our bikes and ride somewhere. Then we'd sit for a while and not say anything. Eventually, one of us would ask, 'So . . . what's up?' That would get us started talking."

Share First

Sometimes if you take the first step by sharing what you're feeling, it can be easier for others to follow. You might say something like, "I'm feeling scared right now. How are you feeling?" Your willingness to let your feelings out can help others feel safe saying what they're really going through.

Be Sure to Check In with Everyone in the Family

It's natural and appropriate for the person with cancer to receive a lot of attention, but it's important to give everyone else in the family the chance to talk about his or her feelings too.

Even though these other family members don't have cancer, they are probably struggling emotionally. For their own health and well-being, everyone in a family affected by cancer needs to have opportunities to talk, vent, or cry. Family members can create such opportunities by asking one another how they're doing.

> "Throughout the time our daughter was receiving treatments, my wife and I made it a point every day to ask our other two children how they were doing. Life was so centered on their sister that we didn't want them to feel lost or forgotten. They were going through a very difficult time too."

> "While Dad was ill, we focused our care and concern almost exclusively on him. It took a while for me to realize that the cancer had overwhelmed Mom, too, and she needed our support. So I made sure to ask her regularly how she was doing during those difficult months. I think she really needed to hear that we were also concerned about her."

> "I was sitting with my sister at the breakfast table before she went to the hospital to see her husband. I asked her, 'How's it going for you?' She was normally stoic, but she began to cry and said, 'This has been even harder than I thought it would be.' Then she described the stress she was under and how it was grinding at her."

"This Is a We Thing"

A survivor told me that once when she was sitting with her husband, he asked her, "How are you doing?" She replied, "Frankly, I'm feeling nervous and afraid, but I didn't want to burden you with any of that." He said, "You don't have to carry this alone. We're walking through this together. This is a *we* thing."

When you ask others how they're doing, it sends a strong message that "This is a *we* thing." It encourages the sharing that can bring family members together.

52

Listen
Carefully

*"My aunt knew that Mom's cancer really hit me hard.
She let me talk whenever I needed to, and she didn't
say much. She let me cry and never said anything like
'You need to toughen up; your mom's the one who's
suffering,' or 'This is the way it is.' She just put
her arm around me and listened."*

As discussed in previous chapters, there will be times when family members would benefit greatly from talking about what they're going through. This is true for both the person with cancer and his or her loved ones. One of the most powerful tools for helping people share is careful listening.

The Qualities of a Careful Listener

Careful listening can encourage sharing, which releases feelings, builds relationships, and brings emotional healing. Here are some characteristics of a good listener.

A careful listener stays focused on the other person. Someone who really listens gives the other person his or her full, undivided attention. Such committed listening shows that the listener greatly values the other person and their relationship. One person told me, "When my kids talked to me about their grandpa's cancer, I made it a point to concentrate on what they were saying and not get distracted by my own internal dialogue. I wanted to hear the real feelings coming from them—not my own thoughts about what they were saying or what I should say next."

When someone listens to you like that, it encourages you to share what's going on deep inside. You know the other person wants to hear what you have to say.

A careful listener shows that he or she is listening. There are a number of ways a person can demonstrate that he or she is listening. The husband of a cancer survivor explained how he did this with his wife: "I would sit close, hold her hand, make eye contact, nod—just do those little things to show I was really engaged in the conversation."

A careful listener asks questions. Asking questions about the other person's thoughts and feelings shows that you're engaged with what he or she is saying, and it invites the person to keep sharing. One woman said, "I'd ask questions to help get at what was going on with my brother and give him space to talk. I'd ask things like 'What do you think about that?' 'How do you feel?' 'What do you think might be the next step?' I didn't tell him what to think or do; I just listened and helped him think it through."

A careful listener pays attention to more than just words. Of course, words are important, but careful listening goes beyond them. One person shared:

> "Mom is so good at picking up on our emotions just from our body language, facial expressions, or tone of voice, looking at more than what's being said. Then she might mention what she's observed—'You're not saying as much as usual; I'm interested in hearing what you're thinking,' or 'You seem really down right now. What's going on?'"

A careful listener encourages the other person to keep sharing. Good listening extends an invitation for the other person to say whatever comes to mind. The sister of a survivor said, "I wanted her to know she could keep talking for as long as she needed to. I kept saying things like 'Yes' and 'Tell me more about that.' Just doing that was enough to keep her sharing for a long time."

A careful listener listens more and talks less. A good listener spends a lot more time listening than talking. Of course, there will be times when it's beneficial to speak, but most of the time it's much more helpful just to listen. One person told me, "My dad would listen and listen and listen. He'd say a few things, mostly to get me to talk, but he'd never cut me off. Afterward, I'd say, 'Thanks, Dad, it was so helpful to talk with you.' And then I'd realize how little he actually said. He knew that *listening* was just what I needed."

A careful listener doesn't try to change a person's thoughts or feelings or solve a person's problems. Good listening isn't about trying to persuade, pressure, or fix—it's about being there and letting the person say what he or she needs to say. A woman shared this example:

"One time I was facing a medical test I knew would be very unpleasant. I said to my husband, 'I don't want this test. I just don't want to do it.' He said, 'I know you don't.' He didn't try to convince me to have the test; he just listened to my concerns and fears. That gave me the freedom to feel what I felt. I did end up getting the test, but I did it because it was what I decided to do."

The Power of Listening

A father told me this story about the relationship-building power of listening:

"I was out walking with my teenage son when my doctor called with the test results: The cancer had not spread! I was crying as I ended the call. I choked out a few words to my son about the good news I had just heard. He looked at me with tears in his eyes and then really listened to everything I said. I didn't have to pretend to be a tough guy—I could show my son my vulnerability and that it was okay to cry. That brought us closer than we'd ever been."

Careful listening is powerful. It promotes the kind of sharing that helps families stick together and stay strong.

53

Create a
Safe Place

*"Mom was always a safe person to talk to. She
would sit with me during treatments or at home,
and I could tell her anything. I could talk or cry or
get upset without fear. She was there for me.
I wasn't alone."*

For honest, helpful sharing to take place, people need to feel safe talking about their deepest feelings and greatest concerns. Families can create a safe place where this kind of sharing can flourish.

What makes the family a safe place to share might be different for each family member and each situation. There may also be situations where a person's safe place involves close friends rather than family. Regardless of the circumstances, a safe place will typically have the following characteristics.

Acceptance

People usually feel safer sharing when they know that the other person will accept what they have to say and not judge, criticize, condemn, or try to fix them. No matter what the person shares, the listener will continue to value him or her and welcome his or her thoughts and feelings.

"My sister never judged me for what I was saying. Whatever I felt—good, bad, sad, afraid, angry, or anything else—she would tell me, 'It's okay to feel that way.' I was free to feel whatever I was feeling and share it with her."

"During our evening walks, I would tell my wife my fears about my father's cancer. She didn't question me, scold me, try to change my thinking, or say, 'Oh no, you shouldn't worry about that.' She welcomed whatever I wanted to say, listened, and let me be me."

Trust

Trust lays a sturdy foundation for safe sharing. In order for people to feel safe expressing their thoughts and feelings, they need to trust that the listener will keep the conversation confidential and respond with care and love.

"My brother became the person I could really count on. We hadn't been very close before, but he visited me right before my surgery, and I just opened up and shared how scared and worried I was. He listened and let me get all those feelings out. We got together regularly throughout my treatment, and I found I could trust him with my deepest fears and concerns. I knew he would keep it all between the two of us. Having someone I could open up to made a huge difference."

"I could trust Dad to be my sounding board whenever I needed to talk about my best friend's cancer. He'd sit beside me, focus all his attention on me, and listen to what I had to say. I felt so encouraged by his presence. Everything he did communicated that I could rely on him."

Honesty

A relationship characterized by honesty can provide a safe place. When you've established that you can be frank with each other, communication can flow more freely. Both of you can say what's on your minds and in your hearts.

"I was diagnosed with cancer shortly after becoming a father, and one of the first things I did was go to see my mother, who had cancer when I was a child. She was candid with me about the fears she'd had as a young mother with cancer. Her honesty helped me to speak up about my own fears."

"My sister and I had been honest with each other all our lives, and my cancer didn't change that at all. I've always been comfortable telling her anything. She'd ask me, 'How are you feeling?' and I could answer truthfully. I knew I didn't have to put on an act with her."

"Right after my husband's diagnosis, we had an honest conversation with our teenage sons. We put everything on the table. We wanted them to know it was okay to be open and up front about their questions and worries whenever they needed to talk."

Genuine Concern

A loved one's heartfelt concern often helps people feel safe. When your words and behaviors express sincere care and a desire to help, they'll provide a warm invitation for the other person to open up.

"I just kept showing up—even when Dad was grumpy after treatments. I never tried to tell him what to do, which he appreciated. I simply listened. I was determined to show him I cared and would always be there for him, no matter what."

"When my mother saw my tears, she would put an arm around my shoulders and say, 'I'm so sorry you have to go through this. Tell me what's going on.' That was my cue to let it all out, knowing she'd care for me all the way through it."

Respect

A safe place is marked by respect. In such a setting, people treat one another as capable and responsible individuals without prying, trivializing others' concerns, or forcing their opinions on others.

"When I told my wife about my uncertainties, she never told me what to think or came at me with her own agenda. She would listen and help me think things through, but she trusted my ability to grapple with these feelings."

"One day, after a particularly hard round of tests, my father listened as I cried and poured out my frustrations. Later, I said to him, 'Thank you for just listening to me and not giving me a pep talk.' It showed that he respected my feelings and didn't want to minimize them."

Privacy

Privacy can help people feel safe sharing. It can be hard to open up when there are others around who might interrupt or overhear, so it may be helpful to provide a setting where you can be alone as you share.

"My wife and I both come from large families, so there were lots of well-meaning people coming and going while she was being treated. I needed to be intentional about making time to be alone with her— taking a drive, walking through the park, making dinner reservations for two. Those were times when she and I both felt at ease to talk."

"I have four sons, and during my treatment they were in middle school and high school. As busy as our family was, if I wanted to talk heart to heart, I needed to set aside time to engage each of them one to one. So I scheduled an occasional 'Mom night' for each of my sons so just the two of us could go somewhere to eat and talk."

No family is perfect. Families sometimes have history that can make it more challenging to share freely and fully. But during the crisis caused by cancer, loved ones may come together in ways they never thought possible to provide mutual care and support. As one person said, "We were no storybook family, but we loved each other through it. When someone needed to share, we went out of our way to provide what he or she needed to feel safe."

Part 9

Relating to Friends and Extended Family

54

Keeping Family and Friends Up to Date

"People cared and wanted to know how I was doing. I updated close family and friends in person or over the phone, but I just couldn't call everyone. So I used the internet to keep most of our friends and relatives informed. It was fast and easy, and it was nice to know they were praying for us and cheering us on."

Your family and friends will undoubtedly want to know what's going on with you and the cancer. Keeping them up to date helps them to stay connected so they can be your best possible supporters.

In chapter 5, "Telling Others about the Cancer Diagnosis," I addressed how to break the news initially. This chapter deals with ways to provide friends and family with follow-up information over time. You'll find a number of ideas here about keeping them up to date. Choose the ones that work best for you.

A good general guideline is to keep others up to date only as much as you want to and are able to. Updating others doesn't have to be a burden; you don't need to give constant, up-to-the-minute reports. Instead, you can keep things manageable by deciding how much you want to share, with whom, and when—and by getting help if you need it.

Ask Someone to Coordinate Your Communications

At times, people may find updating friends and family to be more than they can handle on their own. In those circumstances, it can be helpful to ask a friend or family member to coordinate communications.

Depending on your needs, this person might help with activities such as making and answering phone calls, sending emails, maintaining a personal webpage, or other ways of helping with your communications. Getting help with just some of these activities can free you to focus more of your time and energy on taking care of yourself.

Here are some characteristics to look for in someone who could coordinate your communications:

- Has good communication skills
- Listens carefully
- Follows through
- Is comfortable with whatever tools you decide to use for updating others
- Knows at least some of the people you want to communicate with
- Exercises good judgment about what and what not to communicate and whom to share it with
- Will check with you if he or she is unsure about sharing something

When you choose the right person to coordinate your communications, he or she will be able to take much of that responsibility. It's one less task for you to worry about.

One person told me, "My mother was information-central. I'd check in with her regularly to let her know how I was doing, and she would post updates or handle phone calls with people wanting to know more."

Another said, "My best friend took charge of phone calls, emails, and social media posts. Before sharing any info, he'd check with me about what was confidential and what was okay to tell others, and then he'd make sure friends and family knew what I wanted them to know. Having such a good gatekeeper was a real gift."

If you choose someone to help you by coordinating communications, ask him or her to read this chapter and then discuss what kind of help you'd like.

Update Those You're Closest to in Person or by Phone

It's often good to provide in-person or phone updates for the people you're closest to. Both are personal, reliable ways to stay connected. One person with cancer reflected, "At least some of the time, it helps just to talk to someone about what's going on. Saying it out loud allows the other person to hear you and support you right then and there."

Ways to Keep Extended Family and Friends Up to Date

Survivors and their loved ones have told me about their experiences with the following ways to update extended family and friends.

Email

Some people create email lists and send email updates to a group of people all at once. A family member said, "One advantage of email is that it's immediate. You can quickly send updates to everyone on your list."

Email does have some drawbacks. When you send an email, the recipient can easily forward it to others, and people you never intended might see your communication. So be sure to include only information that you wouldn't mind being shared with others.

Also, as a family member of a cancer survivor said, "You need to think about your audience and know what kind of technology people are used to. My friends, my kids, and even most of my mom's friends have email, but some people in my grandma's generation don't. You need to make phone calls to reach some of them."

Personal Webpage

Websites such as caringbridge.org, carepages.com, and mylifeline.org, as well as some hospital and cancer center websites, provide tools for setting up a personal webpage. There, you can post news about your condition, share photos, request help, and keep a calendar with information about your treatment dates and current needs for support. These websites also offer a place for people to leave personal messages for you.

Many find such a website helpful for updating large numbers of people. A survivor's wife said:

> "Web updates were a piece of cake. I had my computer with me in the hospital and in the chemo room, and I'd update the website to tell people what was taking place. My husband had relatives and friends all over the country, so it was perfect for us."

Another person told me:

> "It got to be exhausting telling people over and over what was going on. Setting up a webpage was helpful because I could type the update once and then a whole group of people could read it. They'd also leave words of encouragement or respond back to help in specific ways. It was a real blessing."

An advantage of updating through a personal webpage is that readers can read as much or as little as they like. One caregiver told me, "Some people wanted every little detail, while others didn't. I put lots of information into my updates for those who wanted to know more, and others could skip the information they really didn't want."

These webpages generally have privacy settings. You can decide whether the information is open to everyone or just to people you invite.

Blog

Some people have updated others by writing a blog. You or a family member might use a blog to share details about the cancer and treatment, chronicle your thoughts and feelings about the experience, and pass along whatever information you'd like.

Although a blog may have privacy settings, it tends to be more public than a personal webpage—people outside your circle of family and friends might come across it and start reading and commenting on your posts. That could be an advantage, because you might find kindred spirits who would offer practical ideas and emotional support. On the other hand, some might feel uncomfortable about having details about their personal situation available to people they don't know.

Social Media

Many people use social media to update friends and family on their condition. For those who have dozens or even hundreds of people they want to keep up to date, social media can be an easy and efficient way to share information that others can read at their convenience.

Social media has also helped some people find the support they need. One person told me:

> "Sometimes I'd post something like 'I'm having a bad day today,' and then I'd get 30 responses saying, 'I'm praying for you.' I always felt much better after getting that kind of support."

Another said:

> "I love being able to reach such a wide audience. When you're going through something like cancer, you don't know who is going to read your post. You put your story out there, and maybe it hits home for just one person who replies, 'Wow, I went through that. I understand.' Then suddenly you're connected with a new friend you might not have found another way. It's amazing."

As with email, communicating via social media won't reach everyone. You may need to reach some people by phone or in person.

Privacy is also an issue to keep in mind. It's easy for people to pass your information along to others you didn't intend to share with. So again, post only information you wouldn't mind others making public to a wider audience.

Video Chat

Video chat programs on your computer or mobile device can help you have face-to-face contact with family or friends who live far away. Being able to see one another can make your update more personal. Some programs allow you to talk with several people at once; one person I spoke with would schedule regular times to talk simultaneously with multiple long-distance friends and family members.

Phone

The phone can be a good means of communication when you're separated by distance or when you want to update people you can't easily reach through other means. In addition to (or even instead of) making calls yourself, you can enlist family and friends to pass information along by phone. You might even write out what you'd like them to share.

Some people have said they occasionally sent updates to certain individuals by text message. This can be a helpful approach for reaching a few people quickly, but it's not as effective for longer communications or for reaching a wider group, so you'll probably want to use other methods as well.

Factors to Keep in Mind

You may want to take some of the following factors into account as you decide how to update family and friends.

Different Kinds of Updates for Different Groups

As much as you care about your family and friends and want to keep them updated, you might not be able to stay in close contact with everyone. One way to care for yourself while keeping others informed is by updating different groups in different ways.

You may have a small circle of your closest confidants—key people who are most actively supporting and assisting you. They're probably the people you'll share information with more frequently and personally, often through face-to-face conversations or phone calls.

Then there may be a larger circle of family and friends who are fairly close to you but aren't playing as active a role. It may be easiest to keep them up to date by using group emails.

A third, still-wider circle may be acquaintances who are interested in knowing how you're doing. This group could include coworkers, neighbors, or people at your place of worship who want to pray for you. You might use a personal webpage, a blog, or periodic social media updates to keep them informed. You also might put information on your congregation's prayer list.

You can decide who is in which circle and how you want to update them.

Privacy

Also consider your privacy needs—what you would be comfortable sharing and with whom. One person said:

> "When my friend had cancer, his wife posted some pretty intimate details related to his condition. I realize that they were okay with revealing such personal information, especially since they had some control over who had access. But I could never feel comfortable sharing that much."

In addition to protecting your own privacy, be careful what you share about others. While writing about their cancer, people have sometimes disclosed personal or awkward information about family or friends. Before you send out a story that your spouse, child, parent, or friend might not want shared, get his or her permission first.

How Many and How Much?

People affected by cancer may wonder, *How many people do I need to update?* The general guideline from the beginning of the chapter applies: Keep others up to date as much as you want to and are able to. It's okay if you don't update everyone. Find the scope and methods of updating that work for you.

Similarly, how much you share is up to you. You don't need to send out an update whenever you have a piece of news. That can become overwhelming to you and to the people you're updating. Just share at a frequency that you're comfortable with.

Updating family and friends is a great way to stay connected with people who care about you and want to know how you are doing. When people know what you're experiencing, they can provide timely support that meets your specific needs. Find the way of updating that works best for you, and get help if you need it.

55

Some Relationships May Change

"Some friends were not around as much as before, while others reached out to me and became closer. I believe all of them responded the best they could—some just didn't know how. Everyone is different."

A cancer diagnosis can rearrange a lot in your life, including some of your personal relationships.

Some relationships may grow more distant. At times, people may pull back or avoid you because they feel uneasy, upset, or scared, which leaves them uncertain about how to relate with you. Thinking about cancer may make them uncomfortably aware that it could affect them or their loved ones as well, or your situation may bring back troubling memories of other experiences with cancer.

One person told me, "A couple of friends saw us less often. They felt awkward being around us. They simply didn't know how to deal with the fact that I had cancer."

If someone initially pulls away and becomes more distant, the change isn't necessarily permanent. After a while, the person might come around and turn into a close supporter. A survivor's husband said, "One of our friends had a hard time coming to grips with my wife's cancer at first, but we left the door open. Over time, she got past her hesitancy and started visiting with us more often."

You may develop new, close relationships. One person said, "I was surprised by how much help and care I got from people who had been just acquaintances or friends of friends. Some of them were every bit as reliable as my longtime best friends were."

Another told me, "I ended up making several amazing new friends. A woman in my book club, someone I knew only casually, became one of my angels. She wasn't fazed at all by my cancer. We became very close, and we still are today."

Some relationships won't change much, if at all. Many of the people you're closest to will stick with you. As one person put it, "My close friends were shocked by my diagnosis—I was too! But then they rallied around me and gave me their full support. They were as loyal and protective as they'd ever been."

A woman said, "My father's two closest friends stayed close to him. They were avid card players who kept up their weekly game with him throughout his illness. They were true friends; they never made him feel like a burden."

Cancer can bring changes to relationships—some may be welcome, and others may be disappointing. You don't need to blame yourself for any of the changes. When you know that these relationship changes are possible, they can be easier to handle.

56

Seek Listeners, Not Lecturers

"When my mother was diagnosed, she called a friend to tell her about it. She had barely gotten out the word 'cancer' when her friend cut her off. For the next ten minutes my mother didn't have a chance to say anything except 'uh-huh' a few times. Her friend went on and on about her grandmother, her brother-in-law, and people at work who'd had cancer—leaving my mother no time to talk about what was happening."

While you're dealing with cancer, you'll have a lot to talk about—your fears, your frustrations, and the various ups and downs you go through. It's important to be able to express your thoughts and feelings when you need to, so seek out a few good listeners you can share with.

One person who had cancer said, "I had a long-distance friend that I knew I could call any time I needed to talk. It made the tough times a little easier and the burdens a little lighter, knowing I could talk and someone would really listen."

Another told me:

"One day at church, someone asked me how my family and I were holding up. I was tempted just to say 'fine' like I usually did, but I decided to take a risk and answer a little more openly. She responded with such compassion and understanding that I stood there talking for a long time as she listened. Having her full attention made me feel validated and cared for—like I really mattered."

Look for people like that—people who are willing to spend much more time listening to you than talking at you. These good listeners set aside their own thoughts and needs for a while and focus all their attention on you. Of course, they do speak from time to time, but only when they have something relevant to ask or helpful to say. Their listening and caring can make your load easier to carry. Listeners can lift your spirits and strengthen your resolve.

But be wary of people who are more likely to lecture than to listen. They may take over the conversation early on and talk almost nonstop about themselves, or other people who have cancer, or what they think you should do. Or they might seem to listen for a while, but then they steer the conversation in a different direction and don't give you another chance to say what you need to. Although they may have good intentions, their lecturing hurts more than it helps. A survivor told me:

> "An acquaintance came up to me and said, 'I'm sorry to hear about your cancer. How are you doing?' Then, before I could get more than a word out, he launched into telling me how I needed to go to a specific cancer hospital where I would have a much better chance of being cured. Then he told me gruesome details about all the people he knew who'd had cancer. As far as he was concerned, it was like I was no longer even standing there. I certainly *wished* I were no longer standing there."

Another said:

> "There were a few friends who constantly voiced strong opinions about what I should or shouldn't do. I suppose they meant well, but their pushiness just upset me. On the other hand, those friends who put my well-being first, who simply listened and offered love and concern, put my mind at ease."

Because you're the one dealing with cancer—your own or your loved one's—it's your right and a healthy choice to spend your time with people who will listen to you when you need to talk. As one person put it, "Being lectured at causes me to shut down, but when someone listens to me, it helps me open up and get my pain out."

When it comes to expressing your thoughts and feelings, you'll benefit most from people who will listen, not lecture.

57

Find One or Two Triple-A Friends

"With most friends, I could share many of my feelings about the cancer, but if I let it all out, the conversation would just shut down. Thankfully, I was blessed with a couple of friends who would allow me to share everything I was experiencing— the good, the bad, and the ugly."

A friend who lives in another city called me during a particularly difficult time in Joan's fight with cancer. When I answered the phone, the first thing he said was, "So how's the *$@#!%, &#?$*! cancer?" (I'll leave his exact choice of words to your imagination.)

By putting it so bluntly, he invited me to say anything I wanted. I knew that no matter what I told him, he wouldn't cringe, judge, or admonish me. He was ready to hear me and accept my full, unfiltered thoughts and feelings, whatever they were.

In addition to finding good listeners as described in the previous chapter, you also may want to find one or two people like my friend—people with whom you can share anything on your mind, everything in your heart. I call these people "Triple-A Friends" because they *Accept Absolutely Anything* you need to share.

When you're talking with Triple-A Friends, you don't need to sanitize your thoughts or filter your feelings to avoid making them uncomfortable. You don't have to pretend to be in good spirits, either. If you feel awful, you can let them know exactly how awful. Whatever you have to say, you can trust these people to handle it without flinching, falling apart, or scolding you for being negative.

Here's what some people told me about having Triple-A Friends:

"I would edit my words when talking to most people. But with one of my friends, I knew I could tell him anything. It was so important to have someone I could share all my painful thoughts and feelings with, and he would just listen and accept me."

"Once, when I was having a really rough time with my treatment, I visited with my friend and rattled off the experiences of the day. She listened to everything I had to say. By letting me voice my hurt, frustration, and fear, she helped me hold body and soul together."

"My friend made it a point to stop in regularly to visit and play board games—and to listen and comfort me. She was the only one I could talk to about my fear and pain. I didn't want to burden my family with that on top of everything else they were dealing with, but she was able to take it."

"Caring for my mother and trying to keep everything together took a lot out of me. One evening, my husband sat next to me on the couch and said, 'Just let it out.' So I did. I cried, I yelled, I poured out my deepest worries. And he just listened and held me. I'd been so busy being there for everyone else that hadn't realized how much I needed someone to be there for me."

"I felt safest talking to my brother. Even though he lived clear across the country, he gave his time freely over the phone. I could tell him anything, and I didn't have to be afraid that he'd judge or reject me. He was always there for me, and he was so supportive."

A cancer survivor I know talked about how, when she was at her lowest point, she found her Triple-A Friend in a Stephen Minister—a trained lay caregiver at her congregation.[1] She said:

---

1 For information about Stephen Ministers, go to stephenministries.org.

"Even though I had friends and family who were eager to care, they just wanted so desperately to see me not hurt. It was easier to put on a happy face and tell them, 'Everything is all right.'

"But whenever my Stephen Minister came to visit me, I could ask all the 'why me?' questions. I could hurt, be afraid, get angry, cry—and know that it was all okay. She didn't try to make it better or tell me what I should do or how I should feel. She just listened and cared."

While dealing with cancer, you'll likely draw on the support of many different people who will help you in many different ways. Be especially on the lookout for one or two Triple-A Friends who will give you the gift of total acceptance and take whatever you throw their way. And when you find someone like that, just let it all out.

58

Tell Others
What You Need

*"My friends welcomed the chance to lend a
hand when I let them know what I wanted—
grocery shopping, driving me to a treatment,
bringing a meal, watering my garden, filling my
bird feeders, or just chit-chatting about life."*

Once word gets around about the cancer diagnosis, family and friends may offer to help. It's uplifting and heartwarming when someone sincerely asks you, "What can I do?" These people are eager to lighten your load, and their practical support can be a lifeline for you.

You can help others help you by telling them what specific kinds of assistance you need. Otherwise, you might end up with ten casseroles sitting in your freezer when what you really need is someone to go with you to treatment or pick up your kids from school on certain days.

Initially, it may feel awkward asking others for help. But this is a time when you really can use assistance, and there are probably people around you who will gladly lend a hand once they know what you need. They'll also appreciate the opportunity to do something to make your life a little easier—it gives them the chance to feel like valued supporters.

One survivor told me, "I've always had a hard time asking for help. But when a friend said, 'Please let me show you how much I care,' I realized how much it meant to others to be able to pitch in. It helps me, and it helps them too."

Determine the Kinds of Help You Need

The first step is to decide what kinds of help you need. People dealing with cancer have told me they appreciated assistance in areas like these:

- Meals
- Caring for children
- Household chores and yard work
- Transportation, especially to and from appointments
- Taking notes during appointments
- Shopping or running errands
- Caring for pets
- Making or answering phone calls
- Keeping extended family and friends up to date
- Researching information about cancer
- Organizing medical information
- Coordinating offers of help from various people
- Just visiting and chatting

You may want to keep a list of your needs and who has offered specific kinds of assistance (or ask someone to help you keep such a list). That way, if somebody asks how he or she can help—or if you need something in particular—you can just check your list. A survivor said, "Sometimes when people asked how they could help, my mind would just go blank. But when I started writing it all down, I could be sure about what I needed. That was a way for me to feel more in control."

Communicate Your Needs

Once you've determined what needs you have, you can share them with people who want to help. Be as specific as you can. If you need a ride at 1:30 P.M. on Friday, say so. If you need meals prepared in a certain way, spell that out. If necessary, you can also enlist someone's assistance in communicating your needs to others. People want to know how to help you, and they'll be especially happy to know they're doing something you really need and appreciate.

One man described how he loved milkshakes and how they were also one of the foods he could keep down most easily while on chemotherapy. When a friend asked about ways to help, the man said he would enjoy having a milkshake. After that, his friend brought him a milkshake whenever he visited. Specifically communicating a need led to a simple way of helping that made both men feel better.

A woman with cancer said it was difficult for her to ask others for help; it just wasn't in her nature. Then one day she mentioned to a visiting friend how much it bothered her that her typically tidy house was such a mess. With the woman's permission, her friend brought another friend along to clean the house the next Saturday. "I quickly learned that people sincerely do want to help," the woman said. "It was just a matter of letting them know what I needed."

Another woman shared:

> "I got the word out about days and times I needed someone to take me to my radiation and chemotherapy appointments. Some of the people who volunteered were unexpected—I didn't have especially close personal relationships with them, but they were eager to help. It touched me deeply to know that so many people cared about me."

These needs don't all have to be practical. If you want companionship or just someone to have some fun with, by all means let people know. One person said, "I love watching comedies on TV, and it's always better with someone else there laughing beside me. One of my coworkers was delighted to come over and watch TV with me. Laughing together was a normal moment in the midst of the not-normal of cancer."

Tell People What You Don't Need

It's also important to let people know the kind of help you *don't* need. A woman whose husband had cancer told me:

> "One area I didn't need help with was cooking. I love to cook, and preparing my family's meals was a way for me to stay in control, so I let people know that I didn't need them to bring us meals. Areas we did need help with were yard work, household chores, and an occasional night out with the guys for my husband. I let people know what we did and didn't need, and they were very happy to help."

Communicate Changing Needs

Needs change over time. Something that's necessary right now might not be as important later on. You might have a greater need for meals one week, housework the next, and childcare or transportation a few weeks after that. Sometimes you may need a lot of help; other times you may need just a little. Communicate your changing needs to others.

Here's an example from one man's experience:

"During my treatment, my brother drove me to appointments, took care of the lawn, and offered general support around the house. After my treatment was completed, I mostly needed to feel in control again and live my life as normally as I could. So I told him how much I appreciated everything he had done but that I no longer needed all that help. He understood but stayed in close contact just in case any other needs came up."

A Win-Win Situation

You probably have people around you who really want to help but aren't sure how. When you describe exactly what you need, many people will be more than willing to pitch in—and grateful for the opportunity.

It's a win-win situation. You get the kinds of help that matter most to you, and your friends get to help you in ways they know will make a difference.

59

Seeing Other People Go On with Their Lives

"Sometimes it was tough to watch other people enjoying themselves while I was sick. I felt cheated. I'd think, 'Why me?'"

Sometimes people with cancer, as well as those close to them, find it difficult to watch others going on with life as usual while cancer fills their own lives with restrictions. They see people around them living normally and happily—going on vacations, attending parties, having a good time, or even just going about their everyday routine—and they think, *I could be doing the same thing if it weren't for this cancer.* The feelings that come with such thoughts can be painful.

Many people with cancer and their loved ones have thoughts and feelings like these. Some people don't have them, but if you do, know that you're not alone—and that it's all right to have them.

Here's how some people described their thoughts and feelings:

"The first time my wife and I went out to lunch after my initial visit with the oncologist, I couldn't bear to watch others relaxing and enjoying themselves at the restaurant. I wanted so badly to be in their place."

❧

"Dad was bedridden for a while during treatment. Once, while a neighbor was taking the trash out to the curb, Dad saw him out the window and said, 'Man, I wish I could do that.' It was hard seeing him wish he could do something as mundane as taking out the trash."

～

"I wanted to get back on the golf course. Before I was diagnosed, I'd just started golfing with my sons, and we were bonding over it. It was so frustrating to hear others talking about golf, because I wanted to be out there playing too."

～

"It was difficult to be together with friends when they started talking about their future plans—trips, graduations, anything. I couldn't make any plans right then. For me, life was in limbo."

～

"My wife would encourage me to go to the kids' football games, school outings, and other activities that she couldn't attend because of her treatment. It was hard for me to see other families with both parents in the stands."

～

"Everything was wonderful for my husband and me. Then the cancer hit, and on some days he couldn't even get out of bed. I'd get angry when I saw couples enjoying anything normal. There was no longer any normal in our lives."

I've talked with many other people who have thought and felt the same way. Keep in mind that such feelings aren't good or bad—they just are. A good way to make those feelings less painful is to acknowledge and express them with a close family member or perhaps a Triple-A Friend.

So, if you experience difficult feelings when you see others doing what you once could do but can't right now, don't feel bad about having those emotions. Just go ahead and feel them.

60

Say No

"I had a lot of trouble telling people no—until I had cancer. That changed my perspective. I needed to protect my time to rest, recover, and just be myself. Saying no helped me feel like I was in control of my life."

When you're dealing with cancer, it helps to set clear boundaries so you can focus your time and energy on taking care of yourself or your loved one and living life fully. For that reason, *no* is one of the most important words in your vocabulary.

From time to time, people may make requests of you, or they may extend an invitation or offer to help you in some way. If you want to say yes, by all means do so, but it's all right to say no if you don't feel up to it or if you aren't interested. Even if the person is proposing something you would ordinarily like to do—such as going to lunch or a movie—if the activity isn't right for you at that time, you can say no without feeling guilty. This principle holds true throughout your life, but it's especially important when you're dealing with cancer.

Here are a few examples of situations in which you might want to say no:

- Someone offers to stop by and chat, but you aren't up to having visitors.

   You can tell the person that this isn't a good time for a visit, adding (if it's true) that you'd be glad to have his or her company another time.

- A neighbor invites you to a barbecue when you are tired and need to stay home.

   You can thank the person for the offer and say that you would love to be there, but this time you need to decline and rest.

- An acquaintance calls to ask whether you'd be willing to talk to a support group about your experience with cancer, but right now you wouldn't feel comfortable talking about it to an audience.

  You can thank the person for thinking of you but say that you aren't ready at this time to talk to an audience about your experience.

- You've been a volunteer for your neighborhood block party for many years, and a neighbor asks whether you'd like to help with this year's event, but you just don't feel up to it.

  You can tell your neighbor that you need to say no to helping out this year so you can focus your energy on getting better.

- You and your child have been invited to a birthday party where there will be many children. You're in the midst of chemotherapy, and your immune system has been weakened.

  You can tell the host that your child would be delighted to come with your spouse but that you must decline since your immunity is down.

Saying no can be challenging. Some people may worry that the person they're saying no to will feel angry or hurt. Others may not believe they have a right to say no. Still others may think that if they decline something—especially when they would have accepted before cancer—they'll be letting cancer control their life, so they end up saying yes and pushing themselves too hard.

Here are some suggestions for how to say no.

Say no simply and politely. You don't have to give lengthy explanations, apologize profusely, or make a big deal about declining. Just offer a simple and polite "no, thank you," along with a brief explanation. Here's an example: "I really appreciate your offer to have us over for dinner on Friday, but I have a treatment scheduled that day, and we're planning to have a quiet evening in. We'd love to do it another time, though." If you would welcome future offers from the person, say so. You might even suggest something else that you would appreciate.

Repeat your no as many times as necessary. If the person doesn't accept your first no, say it again—and keep saying no, calmly and kindly, until the other person gets the message. One individual told me, "Sometimes people didn't want to take no for an answer, so I had to stick to my guns. It was helpful to tell them, 'I need to put most of my energy into dealing with cancer, so I just can't handle much else right now.'" Stand by your decision. Don't let someone pressure you into doing something you don't want to do or don't think you can handle right now. Protect and care for yourself by maintaining clear boundaries.

If necessary, ask someone else to say no for you. Given everything else you're dealing with, sometimes you may not be up to saying no yourself. In such cases, ask a family member, a friend, or someone else to say no for you. One woman said, "After surgery, when I wasn't up to seeing anybody, my sister was great about saying no for me. She relayed the message that it wasn't a good time for visitors right then."

Even if you initially said yes to an offer, it's okay to change your answer to no if you need to. Circumstances can change, and you might need to decline a request you'd originally agreed to. A man with cancer told me:

> "One day, a few friends asked me to join them for dinner the coming weekend, and I said I'd be glad to come. When the day actually arrived, though, I was so worn out from my latest treatment that I had to call back and say I really needed to rest and wouldn't be able to make it. My friends understood the situation and said I'd be welcome to join them the next time."

Remember, you're turning down a request, not rejecting the person. You don't need to feel guilty about saying no. You're only saying no to a specific request; you aren't rejecting the person or ending the relationship. You might tell the person how much you appreciate his or her offer, even though you're saying no this time. One person said:

> "During my mother's treatment, her former employer invited her to the company's holiday party. She called to tell him she wasn't feeling up to it yet but that she was thrilled he asked—and she let him know that she would be there for any parties after her treatment was over."

No is an important word for people with cancer and their loved ones. Use it as much as you need to, and don't feel bad for doing so. Saying no is a matter of self-care and self-respect; it's part of how you live your life and stand up to the cancer as best you can. You can say no in ways that show your care and respect for others, and your honest response can actually strengthen healthy relationships.

Perhaps the greatest benefit of saying no to some things is that it frees you to say yes to other things—those you are able and genuinely want to do.

61

Say Yes

"After my diagnosis, I became much more spontaneous about accepting offers to do something fun or go somewhere new. I didn't want to miss out on any opportunity to enjoy life."

Saying yes is every bit as powerful as saying no when you're dealing with cancer. While saying no sets appropriate boundaries for what you *won't* do, saying yes opens the door to doing what you really *want* to do, including new possibilities you may not have considered.

If you'd really like to do something and it's possible for you to do it, this might be the time to say yes.

No and yes are two sides of the same coin. When you say no to some requests and offers, you can free up the time and energy to say yes to other opportunities that you really want to pursue. Doing so can lead to more fulfillment and enjoyment from life.

One person told me, "Saying yes to things that sounded appealing gave me a newfound burst of energy. It was a chance to take my mind off the cancer and have some fun."

As you're able, you might say yes in situations like these:

- Some friends invite you and your spouse to spend the weekend at a bed and breakfast in a nearby small town. You've always wanted to do that but never gotten around to it. Now, though, you decide to go.

- Normally, you haven't done a lot on your birthday—you've preferred to just spend a quiet day with your family. But when some friends say they'd like to throw a party for you and invite friends and family to celebrate both your birthday and the completion of your treatment, you think that it might be fun, so you're quick to say yes to the idea.

- As long as you've lived in your town, you've never actually taken the time to visit the local art museum. But when you hear that it's going to feature a limited-time exhibition of works by an artist you really like, you decide to check it out.

- You're just about to start a week-long vacation driving up the Pacific coast to admire the beautiful scenery. At the car rental counter, the agent asks whether you'd like to upgrade to a convertible. You haven't driven a convertible before, so after a moment's thought, you say yes.

- You've tinkered around with songwriting for years, and you wished you knew more about how to write a really good song. A friend forwards an email to you about a free online songwriting course being taught by a professor at a famous music school. You've passed up chances to take such classes before, but this time you sign up.

- A local racetrack offers the chance to ride in a racecar with a professional driver. You've been wondering what that would be like, so you go for it.

- The touring company of your favorite Broadway musical is playing a limited engagement, and you go with your spouse to see it. Three days later, someone offers you free tickets to go see the musical again that week. Because you and your spouse really love the show, you accept the tickets and go.

Saying yes to opportunities—when you really want to and you feel up to it—can be a great boost for your enjoyment of life. One person put it this way: "Whenever I can now, I say yes to experiences that sound enjoyable but that I may have passed up before. If I think I can handle it, I jump at the chance to add some zest to my life!"

If the prospect of saying yes to something makes you light up inside, then go for it!

62

Ignore Raised Eyebrows

"My husband and I were late for a connecting flight, and we were hurrying through the airport to the next gate. I could feel my wig flopping as I rushed down the concourse, and I was really sweating. I was so hot that I finally said, 'Oh, what the heck!' I yanked off the wig, stuffed it into my tote bag, and just kept on hustling as if it were the most natural thing. I saw some people do a double take as I hurried by, but I didn't care."

During an extended hospital stay, Joan really wanted to get out for a while. Although she had a nasogastric tube sticking out of her nose, she was able to leave the hospital for a few hours. In that small window, Joan chose to do what always made her feel better—she went to get a manicure.

Now, walking into the salon with a tube in her nose might have raised a few eyebrows, but Joan didn't let that get in the way of doing what she knew would make her feel better.

From time to time, people may raise their eyebrows at what you do. They may stare, shake their heads, or in some other way express their surprise or disapproval over your actions. Don't worry about their reactions. If you want to do something and you're up to it, go ahead and do it.

When you're dealing with cancer, it's perfectly okay to focus on what *you* want and need—on what will make you happier or more comfortable—so long as you respect others' rights. If some people are thrown off by your behavior, that's okay. One person told me, "I used to worry more about what people would say, but cancer changed that. I started focusing on enjoying life, not what others thought!" Another said, "Why restrain yourself out of fear of a few stares or snickers? I was determined to live my life the way I wanted."

You know better than anyone what your needs are and what will make you happy. One person said, "When my mom was in treatment, some people thought she needed to curtail her weekly square dancing. But square dancing is her passion, and she had her doctor's blessing, so she wasn't about to give it up, even when she was wearing a cowgirl hat to cover her bald head."

I know a man who was weakened by chemotherapy but got an okay from his physician to attend the annual campout with his son's Cub Scout pack, as long as he slept in a nearby motel instead of a tent. Most of the other fathers thought this was great, but a few muttered things like, "What's he doing here in that condition?" The man ignored the raised eyebrows and had a wonderful weekend with his son.

Another man shared:

> "My brother loved taking road trips in his motorhome. When he couldn't travel because of his treatment, he still kept the motorhome stocked and ready to go. We would climb aboard, and he'd sit in the driver's seat. He'd say, 'Where do you wanna go today, bro?' and I'd say, 'I dunno, where do you wanna go?' And we would sit out there with the windows rolled down, laughing and pretending we were going on a trip. The neighbors gave us strange looks a couple of times, but we didn't care what they thought."

You have every right to be yourself, no matter how quirky that may be—and that goes double when you're dealing with cancer. Don't let raised eyebrows keep you from doing what makes you the most comfortable or from coping in ways you need to cope. As one person put it, "Sometimes you just need to thumb your nose at cancer, refuse to let it hold sway over you, and keep on being you, no matter what other people may think."

Let others think what they want. Live your life with gusto. Feel free to do what brings you joy or helps you feel more in control. Ignore raised eyebrows and let a little more comfort and happiness into your life.

63

Avoid Toxic
Individuals

*"There was one person who used to come by,
supposedly to show support, but who would actually
dump all her problems on me. Every time she left, I
felt really down and robbed of energy. So I asked her
to stop coming. As someone with cancer, I needed
support and kindness, not stress and irritation."*

As you deal with cancer, there's a chance you may encounter one or more toxic people—individuals who consistently relate to you in hurtful ways.

Toxic people increase your stress, add to your problems, poison your spirit, and make your life even more difficult. Sometimes their behavior can even drive away truly helpful, caring people whose support you need.

Hopefully, you won't encounter any people like this. Nevertheless, it's helpful to know how to spot toxic people and deal with them, in case you come across one.

Warning Signs of Toxic Individuals

Here are some behavioral red flags that can alert you to toxic people. They've probably displayed at least some of these traits all along, but especially after a cancer diagnosis—your own or a loved one's—what they say and do can really make your life miserable.

They are intrusive. Toxic people regularly violate your personal boundaries, use up your time and energy, and push themselves on you even when you make it clear that you need to rest or would prefer to be alone. A survivor told me, "A person I knew called to ask if it was okay if he dropped by, and I said I was having a rough day and wasn't really up to visitors. An hour later, the doorbell rang, and there he was—and he even brought a friend along! I couldn't believe it."

They talk incessantly without giving you much of a chance to say anything. They rarely let you speak, and when they do, it's never long before they jump back in and dominate the conversation again. One person shared her experience: "A friend of a friend came over and asked me, 'What do you really need right now?' I said, 'I just need to talk about it.' She totally ignored what I'd said and started talking nonstop, not even giving me a chance to jump in. It wore me out just listening to her."

They give unsolicited advice and tell you what to do. They assume that they know what's best for you, discounting any responses that don't line up with their advice.

They try to pressure you into being positive. Toxic individuals insist that anything other than perfect cheeriness is unacceptable, making it difficult for you to express your honest thoughts and feelings.

They constantly pump you for information. They pepper you with questions and press you to tell them more, even when you make it clear that you don't want to share. They are more interested in having inside information than they are in caring for you.

They are manipulative and controlling. These people try to work their way into every corner of your life, seize the reins, and take over.

They repeat empty platitudes or make judgmental statements that hurt you or make you feel bad. Any of us may mess up and use unhelpful clichés from time to time, but toxic individuals constantly hammer you with insensitive, hurtful pronouncements.

They are negative and communicate that they expect the worst to happen to you. They may share horror stories in great detail, leaving you anxious or frightened. Their negativity can make you feel exhausted, discouraged, and fearful.

They push unrealistic comparisons on you. They may pummel you with story after story about people who breezed through treatments or always maintained a saintly attitude. Such comparisons can be discouraging or depressing.

Somehow, everything always seems to be about them. Toxic people try to use your cancer to make themselves look good—so they can feel heroic and others will think they're coming to your rescue. As one person said, "These people live for drama, and they want a starring role in your life so they can say, 'Look at me! See what a wonderful person I am!'"

Now, it's important to distinguish between occasional toxic behavior and a toxic individual. Any of us may blunder and behave in an unhelpful or even hurtful way every once in a while. That doesn't make us toxic—just human. Truly toxic individuals, on the other hand, engage in some or all of these behaviors regularly, predictably, and to an extreme. These are people you're better off just not dealing with.

The Painful Effects of Toxic Individuals

Here's what some survivors and their loved ones have told me about their experiences with toxic people:

> "I had to keep my distance from one self-centered relative because after every conversation with him, I felt like I'd just run a marathon and then gotten run over by a truck. I flat-out told him to stay away."

> "One acquaintance always grilled me for details and regularly predicted doom and gloom. One day when I was feeling fine, she came up to me and said, 'Your color is off; you look sick. Are you all right? You'd better lie down.' It was rude and uncaring. I realized she didn't care how I was really doing; she just reveled in my suffering. I had to tell her to knock it off—I didn't want to hear any more of it."

> "My wife had a strained relationship with an uncle. He was so negative that she would always feel a bit sicker after she got off the phone with him. Whenever he called, I'd get stressed out because I knew how his calls hurt her. Finally, we decided that whenever we saw it was him on the caller ID, we wouldn't take the call. We both felt a lot better."

"There were a couple of people I just had to stay away from. I called them 'energy-suckers' because *they* left feeling satisfied and rejuvenated, while *I* felt like they'd sucked the life out of me. When you're dealing with cancer, the last thing you want or need in your life is energy-suckers."

"One day when I arrived at my mother's house to take her to the doctor, I found her in tears because a woman had just spent two hours telling her everything that could go wrong. My mother told me that the woman did this to her every time she visited. So I called the woman and disinvited her from visiting or calling my mother from then on. I didn't feel a bit guilty, because my mother was already fighting an uphill battle. She didn't need someone pushing her down again and again."

How to Deal with Toxic Individuals

Unfortunately, toxic individuals generally don't grasp how self-centered and hurtful their behavior can be. Because of this, the best solution for dealing with toxic people is to set boundaries and, as much as possible, refrain from relating with such individuals. Don't call them or invite them to visit you. Don't take their calls. You have every right to do this. You are under no obligation to spend time with people who hurt or discourage you.

If setting boundaries is difficult for you, ask a family member or friend to deal with any toxic person who writes, calls, or shows up unannounced. Show this chapter to those helping you so they'll understand your need for this kind of help. Anyone who's willing to help you in this way is a true friend. One person told me, "Sometimes problems can be stopped before they start. I ran interference for my mother, and it made things a lot easier for her."

You don't ever have to feel guilty about not relating to toxic people. That's true at any time, but especially when you're dealing with cancer. As one survivor said, "This is your life; this is a time to focus on you. Surround yourself with people who lift you up, and distance yourself from those who drag you down. Your health and well-being are more important than whatever they want from you."

When you realize that someone has a toxic effect on you, it's perfectly all right to distance yourself from that person. You'll preserve your energy, protect your peace of mind, and provide yourself with more time for life-giving people and activities.

Part 10

Additional Support

64

Find
Kindred Spirits

"I'm especially close to two others who also have cancer. The three of us are like a team. We pass along what we've learned. We cheer each other on. We laugh, cry, and share together. We understand each other. It really helps me to know others who have similar thoughts and feelings."

When I travel, I often see military personnel flying from one place to another. I'm always impressed by the way they relate to one another—how they greet each other, chat, and laugh together. There's an unmistakable bond between them. They are kindred spirits because they've been united by a significant, shared life experience.

You may form the same sort of connections with others who have experience with cancer—people who have walked a path like yours.

One woman told me about the many ways she was blessed by such a kindred spirit:

"I first met my friend in the waiting room just before an appointment with my oncologist. She was a stranger at the time, but she and I struck up a conversation right away. When I was called in for my appointment, she gave me her number so we could continue our conversation later. We formed an instant friendship that grew as time went on.

"She was three months ahead of me in treatment, so she helped me mentally prepare for the ups and downs ahead. She would encourage me, and I would encourage her. We felt safe opening up to each other and could serve as sounding boards for each other's feelings.

"Now, 18 years later, we're still such good friends that my husband jokingly says we must be attached at the hip. The two of us have formed a deep bond of sisterhood that was vital throughout the cancer—and beyond!"

How to Find Kindred Spirits

You might be surprised at how often you encounter kindred spirits without even going out of your way to search for them; they can show up in places and ways you wouldn't expect. One man told me, "I had asked to be included in the Sunday prayers at church. After the service, several men came up and told me they were cancer survivors, and it turned out that two of them had the same kind of cancer that I did." A woman said, "When I went wig shopping, I saw another woman looking at wigs—a complete stranger—and started talking with her. We didn't stay strangers for long. Our shared experience led to a lasting friendship."

You also may want to actively seek out kindred spirits. One man said, "When I found out I had colon cancer, I made a beeline to my brother-in-law, who'd had it a few years before. He freely shared his time and experiences with me, and I developed a deeper connection with him."

If you don't know anyone who could qualify as a kindred spirit, you might ask your medical team, your pastor, your family and friends, or someone else to point you in the right direction. A survivor shared with me, "I was about to start treatment when I asked a friend whether he knew someone I could talk to. He mentioned that six months earlier, his son-in-law had completed the same treatment. I got in touch with him, and he was very helpful in giving me an idea of what to expect."

Benefits of Kindred Spirits

There are two important benefits of finding kindred spirits.

Mutual Support

The first benefit is mutual support. You'll be able to offer each other empathy and understanding that you can't often get from someone who hasn't dealt with cancer. There are times when you just need to talk with someone who really understands what you're going through. Kindred spirits are great for that.

One person said:

"It was a relief when I could let my guard down and be honest with someone. Since we were both going through this, we understood each other on a level that others could not. We built each other up during low times and celebrated together during good times."

Another told me:

"At first, my mother was so frightened about chemotherapy, and nothing we said seemed to help. But at her first treatment, she ended up sitting next to a little girl with leukemia who had received several treatments already. The girl told her, 'It's okay to be scared—I'm scared too—but you can be a *big girl* just like me!' In her treatment sessions that followed, Mother had several conversations with her new little friend and always looked forward to seeing her. None of us could calm Mother's fears the way that young girl could."

Sharing What You Learn

The second benefit is sharing what you're learning about handling various challenges. Kindred spirits are people with whom you can exchange tips, pass along ideas, or talk about what you've found out. You'll learn much more quickly as you each share what you've picked up or experienced.

One man shared, "I connected with someone who had the same kind of cancer I had. We talked about how we handled different issues that came up, including some that I wouldn't have felt comfortable talking about with most people." A woman said, "I got all kinds of practical tips from my friend. I felt more prepared and more in control of my out-of-control situation."

Kindred Spirits for Loved Ones

The loved ones of someone with cancer can benefit from kindred spirits too. I discovered several after Joan was diagnosed, and I got to know two of them very well. Both were men whose wives were also being treated for cancer.

I met one of them in the waiting room during our wives' treatment. We got to talking, and when we realized how similar our experiences were, we decided to stay in contact.

I met the other man at a conference; he's the person I mentioned in chapter 15, "Network with People Who Have Been There." This was a long-distance friendship—he lived on the East Coast, and I was in St. Louis—but we were able to stay in touch by phone and email.

Both relationships were invaluable sources of support and information as we traveled on our separate but similar journeys.

When you find a kindred spirit, you've found a special ally. Not only can you share what you are learning, but you can also give and receive a unique level of understanding and moral support along the way.

65

Consider a
Support Group

*"One of the best things I did was join a
support group where we all shared our feelings and
experiences. Cancer can be isolating, so participating
in that group was very helpful for me."*

Cancer can leave people feeling lonely. Cancer support groups connect those affected by cancer with others who have faced or are facing many of the same challenges and choices.

What Happens in a Support Group?

In a cancer support group, people dealing with cancer gather to share experiences, provide mutual care, and talk about their fears and hopes.

There are different types of support groups, such as:

- groups open to anyone dealing with any kind of cancer
- groups for those with a particular type of cancer
- groups for those with a particular stage of cancer
- groups for family members of those with cancer

Each support group has a facilitator or moderator who guides the discussion and keeps the group focused. Some groups are led by a professional such as a social worker, oncology nurse, chaplain, or counselor. Others have a lay facilitator, often a cancer survivor.

Regardless of the type of group, the purpose is *support*. These groups are gatherings where people encourage and comfort one another while also sharing insights for coping with the physical and emotional aspects of cancer.

Benefits of Support Groups

Support groups can offer a variety of benefits to people with cancer and to their loved ones:

- Support groups connect you with people who have had experiences similar to what you're going through—people who can offer empathy and understanding. One person described it this way: "It helps me to be around other people who've had some of the same thoughts and fears I have. They better understand what I'm facing because they've been there themselves." Another said, "The others in my support group treated me like a regular person. That was so refreshing after dealing with some people who seemed to think of me only as 'the person with cancer.'"

- Support groups can give you a safe place to talk about your difficult feelings or let off emotional steam. A survivor told me, "I was able to speak freely in my support group. I could tell them things that might have upset my family and friends."

- People in the group can share practical information—useful tips that might make your life a little easier.

- Even if you're not comfortable telling others what you're going through, you may benefit just from hearing other people talk about facing similar challenges.

- You may gain hope and reassurance, as was the case with a woman who told me, "Several people in my support group are longtime survivors—they've fought this disease and beaten it. Talking with them energizes me with hope that I can beat this too!"

You may find a support group helpful whether or not you already have supportive family and friends. One person told me, "I had a lot of support from my immediate family, but I still got a lot out of my group." Another said, "I was single and had recently moved across the country, so when I was diagnosed, I was basically alone. I joined a support group, and they became my nearby family and friends."

That being said, support groups won't appeal to everyone. Some people prefer not to participate in one. A number have told me they simply aren't wired that way, or they found all the support they needed elsewhere. What matters is that you draw on the type of support that feels right to you.

Finding the Right Group

You can find support groups in a number of ways, such as asking your oncologist and others on your medical team, contacting the American Cancer Society or another cancer organization, or searching online. Many hospitals and treatment centers sponsor support groups, as do some churches and counseling centers. You might also learn about support groups as you network with others who are dealing with cancer.

Once you've identified a support group that you may want to try, it's helpful to contact the leader of the group to learn more. Based on that conversation, you can decide whether you'd like to visit and try it out.

Getting Started in a Group

You may want to attend two or three meetings of a particular group before deciding whether to participate in it long term. That way, you'll have a better feel for the group and the people in it. Some have found it helpful to bring a family member or friend to those initial meetings.

Each support group is unique, with its own blend of people, purpose, process, and personality. If one group doesn't feel right, you may want to try another group to see whether it's a better fit.

Also consider whether it's the right time for you to be in a group. If you try one or more groups and they just don't work for you, you may want to try again after some time. It could be that you're not quite ready now but would benefit later on.

You might get a lot out of a support group, or you might do better with other kinds of support. It's also possible that you'll find a support group to be more helpful at certain times and less helpful at others. What's important is that you find the support you need.

66

Share, Don't Compare

"When I focused on how others had it easier or harder than I did, I was my own worst enemy. I did better when I stopped worrying about differences and just focused on what I was going through."

Whether among kindred spirits, in a support group, in a waiting room, or elsewhere, you'll probably end up talking to a lot of people who have had many different experiences with cancer. When you do, it can help to share with them what you're going through and listen as they share their experiences. It isn't helpful, however, to dwell on comparisons between your situation and theirs.

Sharing involves people talking about their own circumstances and challenges while facing cancer—their highs and lows, their tough decisions, their physical and emotional pain, and what they've learned along the way. Such sharing can do a lot to lighten the load of dealing with cancer.

Comparing happens when people contrast their own experiences with what others are going through—trying to determine whose situation or way of handling things is worse or better. A person may think, *She's suffering more from side effects than I am, so who am I to complain?* or *He and I are receiving the same treatment, so why am I having a harder time?*

Because we're human, comparisons—and the uneasy feelings that can accompany them—seem to come naturally. All of us may find ourselves comparing a little now and then, but dwelling on comparisons can really drag you down. It's better to let go of comparisons, as much as possible, and focus on sharing instead.

One woman told me:

"Treatments really knocked me flat for days, but my friend was able to continue working during her treatment. She even helped plan her daughter's wedding, all while fighting cancer! It just didn't seem fair.

"Eventually, though, I came to realize that we were two different people, each dealing with our own hurts and challenges—it didn't matter whose situation was better or worse. As long as I kept that in mind, I received a lot of comfort from talking with her, and I think she got the same from me."

Here's how a man described his choice to share rather than get caught up in comparing:

"A coworker and I happened to have the same basic type of cancer at the same time, but that was where the similarities ended. We had different surgeries, different medications, different side effects, different timelines, and different paths to a successful outcome. We quickly realized that, with all these differences, comparing our experiences would be a waste of time, so we just focused on supporting each other."

Dwelling on comparisons won't make you or the other person feel any better. So as you relate to others who are also facing cancer, welcome opportunities to share, but avoid the temptation to dwell on comparisons.

67

Be Open
to Professional
Counseling

*"I could let everything out with my counselor. He
listened to all of it and helped me understand that
it was natural to have all these conflicting feelings.
He made it safe to talk about those things
I couldn't share with anyone else."*

Fighting cancer is not only a physical battle. It's also an emotional one, both for the person with cancer and for his or her loved ones. It's only natural for people to wrestle with many difficult feelings while dealing with cancer. Sometimes it's a good idea to get help in handling those feelings, possibly from a professional counselor.

Professional counselors—which include psychologists, psychiatrists, psycho-oncologists, clinical social workers, psychiatric nurses, pastoral counselors, and others—are trained to help people identify, understand, and manage life's challenges. Counselors assist people in finding the most effective ways to respond to crises. They remain focused on the individual and his or her needs, helping the person work through tough times. They provide care, wisdom, and support while remaining impartial and objective. Counselors keep what people share with them strictly confidential. They're trained to be nonjudgmental listeners, so people can let it all out.

If you think you might benefit from professional counseling, talk with your medical team. They can help connect you with counselors who have experience working with cancer patients and their loved ones.

Counseling Can Benefit Anyone

I want to clear up one common misconception: Professional counseling is *not* just for people dealing with serious mental health issues. It's also beneficial for anyone who is simply feeling overwhelmed. One person said, "At first I balked at the suggestion of counseling. I thought it was for people with severe emotional problems. But a trusted friend assured me that counseling would be appropriate for me, and after I went, I really did feel better. My thinking was clearer, I saw issues for what they really were, and I became stronger." Another described counseling this way: "My counselor gave me a place to dump all my difficult feelings—anger, fear, sadness, despair—so I could get them out of my system. It was freeing to talk about all that I was feeling, knowing I didn't have to filter any of it." Professional counseling can be a great source of support and insight for anyone affected by cancer, both those diagnosed and their loved ones.

Of course, professional counseling is urgently and absolutely needed in some situations, such as when a person is showing signs of severe depression or having suicidal thoughts. In these instances, the person needs help right away.

Counseling Can Benefit Loved Ones

When people receive care through professional counseling, it benefits the people close to them as well. One man told me, "My family was already stretched to the limit trying to meet my physical needs. My counselor provided the focused emotional support I needed, which was a big thing my family didn't have to worry about." A mother whose child was being treated for cancer said, "I went to a psychologist because I was overwhelmed by taking care of my son while trying to hold the family together. Counseling was something I needed for myself so I could be there for everyone else."

Not everyone dealing with cancer needs or wants professional counseling, but if you do, it's important to know that seeking counseling isn't a sign of weakness. Recognizing one's limits and reaching out for help as needed shows real strength and courage.

Part 11

Spiritual Matters

68

The Spiritual
Side of Dealing
with Cancer

*"Cancer forces you to claim what is truly important
to you—including what's important spiritually.
Cancer makes you ask the hard questions."*

Cancer can certainly affect you physically, emotionally, and relationally. But it can also affect you spiritually, touching the core of who you are and what you believe, causing you to ask tough, profound, urgent questions.

- *Why me? Why this? Why now?*

- *How could this happen?*

- *Where can I find hope now that cancer has turned my world upside down?*

- *I feel so alone. Does anyone understand what I'm going through?*

- *Where is God in all this?*

I've talked with people from a variety of faith traditions, as well as people with no faith background, and I've found that it's common for those dealing with cancer to wrestle with what they believe about themselves, their lives, and God. Here's what some of them have told me about their spiritual struggles:

"I was a single mom with two young children when I was diagnosed. I just couldn't understand why God allowed this. Didn't he care about my children? I started trying to make deals with God: 'Please take care of me so I can take care of them.'"

"My family and I have been through many hardships, and my faith has always gotten me through. But when my brother told me he had cancer, I couldn't believe it. He was my best friend. All I could think was, *This shouldn't happen to him, God. Why didn't you prevent this?*"

~

"When my husband was diagnosed, I spent time asking, 'God, how can I go through this—being a caregiver and provider when he was always the one supporting us?' Then I'd feel guilty for even thinking that."

~

"When I told our son about my diagnosis, he was so upset that he went outside, picked up a patio chair, and threw it halfway across the yard. He was very angry with God over how unfair it all seemed."

~

"At the time of my diagnosis, my faith was precarious at best. For a while I thought my cancer must be a cruel punishment, and I asked, 'Why, God? What did I do to deserve this? Why are you doing this to me?'"

~

"At first, it seemed like God had disappeared—I felt nothing. But I must have still believed deep inside. At each turn, I kept meeting God in new ways. I started out in the void, but as I struggled with it, I gradually found a deeper, more hopeful understanding."

Cancer can bring a crisis in matters of faith, whether you have very strong spiritual beliefs, have no spiritual beliefs, or find yourself somewhere in between. A cancer diagnosis can raise a lot of deep concerns and hard, even troubling questions. The next four chapters explore ways to prepare for and address these concerns and questions.

69

A Spiritual
Roller Coaster

"My faith was topsy-turvy as I fought cancer. At times I was angry at God; at times I was grateful for his help; at times I felt abandoned; at times I was filled with hope. I had times of pushing God away followed by times of feeling close to him."

Chapter 3, "A Roller-Coaster Ride," says that dealing with cancer is like riding an emotional roller coaster—one day's news can lead to a sense of relief or even celebration, while another day's results can cause disappointment or frustration.

You may also experience spiritual ups and downs. One day you may think you have satisfactory answers to your deeply spiritual, meaning-of-life questions. But the next day, those answers may be clouded over with confusion or doubt. Then, a day or two after that, the sun comes out, and you see things more clearly again.

There may be times when you're looking for God, and it feels like you're staring into an abyss. Later, you may be surprised by a new, greater awareness of God in the midst of your pain, finding God's love and compassion drawing you close when you're suffering most. After that, the spiritual roller coaster may plunge back down as you ask questions like:

- *Why me?*

- *Why did God allow this to happen to me?*

- *Is this some kind of cruel test?*

- *Why does God seem a million miles away now that I need him more than ever?*

- *Have I lost my connection to God?*

- *I'm frightened and in pain—why isn't prayer helping?*

A number of people have described such spiritual highs and lows in dealing with cancer. One said:

> "The weeks after diagnosis brought huge swings in my faith—from complete trust in God to overwhelming fear that I was all alone. It took time before I believed that God was journeying through this right alongside me."

Another told me:

> "As I prayed for the strength just to get through the day, sometimes it felt like God gave me the help I needed, and sometimes it didn't. There were days when I would seek God's presence and be unable to feel it. Other days I felt surrounded by God's love. The ups and downs left me feeling a bit bewildered."

Anyone may experience these swings. As one pastor put it, "Cancer can rattle even the strongest foundation."

These ups and downs don't happen to everyone, but many people dealing with cancer go through times when they're angry at God, mired in doubt, or feeling abandoned—followed by periods when they connect meaningfully with God, feeling confidence and comfort as they trust that God is with them every step of the way.

70

Be Totally Honest
with God

"As I drove home from the hospital, I yelled at God: 'Okay, enough is enough! This is the last straw. What are you thinking? I can't do this. This is going to break me.' It was probably the most honestly raw moment of my life."

In chapter 57, "Find One or Two Triple-A Friends," I described the kind of person who can give you the gift of complete acceptance. It can be beneficial to search for such a person.

But we also have someone immediately available to us—someone we can share anything with, anytime we need to.

We can be totally honest with God.

People sometimes wonder whether it's okay to be totally honest when they're talking to God. They may worry that they have to watch what they say, or else God will get angry or reject them. So they hold back.

But you *can* safely talk to God about anything you're thinking or feeling—even if you're angry, even if you're having thoughts you aren't proud of, even if you're questioning whether God loves you, even if you're wondering whether God actually exists. You'll never share anything God doesn't already know, and there's nothing you can say that will cause God to love you less. In fact, there isn't anyone safer to share everything with.

A survivor said, "After a while, it hit me: *God already knows what's in my heart and mind—whether or not I express it—and accepts me just as I am. Nothing I say can surprise God.* That was very freeing; I can be angry or disappointed or frustrated and feel free to let it out when I'm talking to God."

In *Don't Sing Songs to a Heavy Heart,* I wrote about holding nothing back with God:

> Does God want to have a relationship with the real you? Or will God be content to have a relationship with some phony, prettied-up, pious you?
>
> This question is posed in such a way that you can't get the answer wrong. God wants the real me, you say. Of course!
>
> If you accept that, then the next question is, *How angry are you allowed to get at God?* How much wailing, screaming, crying, and venting are you allowed?
>
> *As much as it takes* is the answer. *As much as your feelings demand.*
>
> The truth about God here is very clear: God can take whatever you can dish out.[1]

What can you share with God? Anything and everything. You don't need to worry about causing offense or hurting God's feelings. You don't need to filter your words when you talk to God.

If you feel angry, hurt, sad, anxious, afraid, betrayed, or abandoned by God, say exactly what you're feeling. If you're not sure what you believe about God, feel free to express your doubts. When you just don't understand why something has happened, cry out to God. And if you're unsure of what to do or weighed down with a heavy load, ask God for help—even insist on it.

People have been honest with God for millennia. The Bible candidly shows suffering, struggling people bringing their fear, anger, and uncertainty to God. To give just a few examples, there's the story of Job, many of the Psalms, the books of Ecclesiastes and Lamentations, and even Jesus in the garden of Gethsemane and on the cross. So when you honestly tell God what you're thinking, feeling, or needing, you're in good company.

Here's what some cancer survivors and loved ones have told me:

> "I spent hours shouting and shaking my fist at God. I'm so thankful that God can handle my anger, because I was *furious* at times. I told him, 'I've had enough, and I hate the way you're doing things!'"

---

1 Kenneth C. Haugk, *Don't Sing Songs to a Heavy Heart: How to Relate to Those Who Are Suffering* (St. Louis: Stephen Ministries, 2004), p. 72.

"While I was out walking or spending quiet time alone, I would talk with God, asking, 'Why? Where do I go from here? How could this possibly serve you?'"

"After two months of getting angry at others, I realized that I was actually angry with God. This was the first time in my life I could remember having such severe anger toward God. After God and I had a long talk, my emotions finally began to heal."

"It was only when I let it all out to God that I understood how deep his love for me really was."

"Yelling at God seemed outrageous to me. But then, how outrageous is it to have cancer cells attacking your body?"

"When my cancer came back, it seemed so unjust. I was asking God, 'Why? What have I done? Why me? I don't understand what you want from me!'"

"I wasn't always sure if others could handle hearing about what I was really going through. But when I was talking to God, I could be completely honest about my fears for the future and what this cancer was doing to my family. When I shared my feelings with God, I knew I wasn't going through this alone."

So go ahead and tell God everything on your mind and in your heart. Yell at God if you need to. It can be a huge relief just to let it all out, whether you cry out silently inside your head or shout out loud at the sky.

When you need to honestly share all that you're thinking and feeling, it's good to know that the one you're talking to will love and accept you no matter what. That's exactly the kind of love and acceptance God gives us. You don't have to hold anything back from God.

71

Exercise
Your Spirituality

"During the emotional upheaval after my diagnosis, I got into the habit of reading a devotional and saying a prayer every day. As the initial shock wore off, my new habits remained. They anchored me, and the reality of God cut through my fear and brought me peace."

Spirituality is a lot like a muscle: The more you exercise it, the stronger it gets. People from a number of religious traditions told me about ways they exercised their spirituality while dealing with cancer and how they benefited. Here's an overview of spiritual practices that people have found helpful and meaningful. Different practices may be more meaningful for you at different times, so use the ones that are the best fit for you right now.

Prayer

"During radiation treatments, I usually pray as I lie on the table. I pray to be cured. I pray for other patients to be healed. I pray for the doctors and technicians giving the treatment. Praying gives me hope."

"I pray a lot. I talk with God when I wake up in the middle of the night and can't sleep. I write to God about my anger when it wells up. For me, the important thing is to try to stay in communication with God."

"Sometimes my most powerful prayer is just 'Help!'"

Reading the Bible

"I carry a little card with Bible verses written on it to all my treatments. I read them over and over to find the strength to face whatever will come."

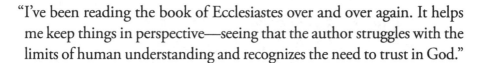

"In the Psalms I've found people who were in pain and feeling abandoned and crying out for God to help them. Their words have become my words too."

"I've been reading the book of Ecclesiastes over and over again. It helps me keep things in perspective—seeing that the author struggles with the limits of human understanding and recognizes the need to trust in God."

"My wife got me an audio recording of the Bible so I can listen to it when I'm too tired to read."

"I go back to the account of Jesus' suffering again and again. It comforts me to know that God understands what I'm going through because of everything Jesus went through. I read all four Gospels, but I like John the best. That's the one where Jesus asks one of his disciples to take care of his mother. It helps me remember that God is also taking care of me."

Worship

"Attending worship services gives me comfort, peace, and hope. Worshiping with others helps me know I am not alone. I feel surrounded by God's presence."

"We attend church every Sunday we can. Even though my husband is thinner and he's lost his hair, he doesn't worry about it. He just wants to go to church."

"When I couldn't go out because my immune system was weak, I would watch the Sunday worship service on my congregation's website. It helped me feel connected to church and to God."

Holy Communion

"Receiving Holy Communion is one of the most powerful ways I connect to God. I feel Jesus right there with me, like I'm on holy ground."

"Jesus said we should remember him when we take communion. I remember him, and I feel hope."

"When I couldn't leave home, a Eucharistic Minister came to my house to serve me communion. Those were times when I most felt God's caring presence, as if God was visiting me in my home."

Meditation

"For me, meditation is a silent time alone when I just close my eyes and allow God's love to embrace me. It's just being present with God."

"Taking time to be quiet and meditate helps me grow closer to God and find some direction for the best way I might serve him when I'm well again. It gives me something hopeful and meaningful to look forward to."

"When I was feeling anxious or overwhelmed, I would sometimes comfort myself by closing my eyes and going through the alphabet, thinking of words that describe God. For example, I'd think, *A—God the Almighty. B—God, who Blesses me. C—God is Compassionate. D—God is my Deliverer.* . . . It helped me keep my eyes fixed on God and filled me with peace and hope."

Spiritual Journaling

"I keep a prayer journal where I write the Scripture verses and messages from the cards and letters I've received, along with the names of the people who sent them. Then I read my journal whenever I'm feeling low, such as on the days of my chemo treatments or scans. It's comforting to see God's messages and the names of all those who are praying for me."

"I learned that psalms of lament start by calling out to God and telling him about your pain, then continue by asking for God's help and strength, and end by praising God. I write my own laments, and it's a powerful experience. Knowing they will end in praise helps me to face the dark places."

Music

"Whenever I visit my mom in the hospital, I play recordings of gospel songs that she really enjoys. I know the healing power of music. It has always been a very important part of our spiritual life."

"I don't have a great voice, but I love music that praises God. So when no one else was home, I would sing out loud. It was energizing to lift my voice to the Lord—it amazed me how much it changed my attitude."

"A friend downloaded some of my favorite inspirational music so I could take it with me and listen to it whenever I wanted to—at home, during treatments, and while I was waiting to see the doctor. The music took me into God's presence and calmed me down when I was feeling stressed."

Nature

"I spend time soaking up the beauty of nature and admiring what God has made. My family even put a bird feeder outside my bedroom window so I could continue to enjoy a bit of nature while I was stuck in bed."

"I feel most connected to creation when I'm out in my garden. I've had to scale back on my gardening during treatment, but it's still my best way to let go of stress and find some peace."

"When I have the energy for it, I love going for a drive out into the wide-open spaces and then taking a walk. Being out in nature renews and refreshes me—I experience how big God is, and it gives me a sense of awe and wonder."

"I like sitting in the sunlight, outside or by a window. The warmth of the sun on my skin feels like God is holding me in his hands."

Devotional Reading

"A friend gave me a devotional book, which I read every night. It calms me and helps me know I'm not alone. God is going through this with me and taking care of my loved ones."

"It isn't always easy for me to just open up the Bible and read it, but a book of daily devotions has really helped. Each devotion gives me a Bible passage to read and explores the meaning of that passage. It's opened my eyes to different ways of looking at God and what's happening to me."

Anointing

"One of my dad's favorite biblical figures is David, and Dad wanted to be anointed like David describes in Psalm 23. So I asked the pastor to anoint my dad with oil and pray for his healing."

"When I was first diagnosed, I told my pastor what was going on, and he offered to anoint my head and hands and ask God to heal me. That's remained a physical sign that God is traveling with me on my journey."

Serving Others

"Service is at the core of my spirituality. It's a way to take my inner fight and turn the energy outward, and it gives me a sense of satisfaction to know that I'm serving God by serving others."

"As I'm able, I keep up with some of my volunteering to maintain some continuity and meaning in my life."

These are just some of the ways you might exercise your spirituality. Find whatever helps you strengthen your spiritual muscles—and keep on exercising!

72

Seek Out Spiritual Community

"As soon as my church family learned about my diagnosis, they were there—praying with me, comforting me, and reassuring me that I wasn't facing this alone. I don't see how I could have made it through this ordeal without them."

Many people dealing with cancer have discovered the benefits of spiritual community, of interacting with others who share similar beliefs. Often, by relating with people of faith, they can experience a closer connection to God and receive comfort, strength, and encouragement. To experience similar benefits, you may want to seek out spiritual community, whether with people you already know or with people who are new to you.

Spiritual community can be found in one-to-one relationships, small groups, or larger gatherings.

One-to-One Spiritual Community

Sometimes you can find spiritual community with just one other person, such as a family member, a friend, a prayer partner, or a spiritual leader.

A Family Member

Your closest spiritual relationship may be with your spouse, a sibling, or another member of your family. A survivor told me, "My husband would hold my hand and read a devotional book to me. It was a time of spiritual intimacy and encouragement for us both."

A Friend

A friend can reach out and provide spiritual care during shaky times. One person said, "After I was first diagnosed, a dear friend came over right away to visit and pray with me. When we talked, I felt comfort, strength, hope, and peace. Her being there helped me understand that God would be with me no matter what."

A Prayer Partner

Having a prayer partner can reduce the challenge of praying and increase the emotional and spiritual support it offers. Your partner might pray *with* you when you're together—and *for* you when you're apart. One person shared, "When my treatments took me out of town, my prayer partner stayed in touch to ask me what to pray for. Several times we even prayed together long-distance via video chat."

You might find a prayer partner at your place of worship or among your friends. A survivor said, "Having a prayer partner has been an incredible blessing. It's someone I can depend on, someone I can trust with all my doubts, fears, and raw feelings. What a wonderful gift!"

A Spiritual Leader

Others have told me how a spiritual leader made a big difference during a crucial time, offering support, understanding, and insight. One woman said, "Within hours after the diagnosis, our pastor was at our home, listening to our fears, praying with us, and anointing my husband. It was just the support we needed right then."

Small-Group Spiritual Community

Besides one-to-one relationships, it's often helpful to seek out a small, close-knit group of people for spiritual community. A Sunday school class, a Bible study group, a church choir, a faith-based small group, a cancer support group organized by a congregation—these are just a few possibilities. One person shared, "When my wife was diagnosed with cancer, we were lucky to be part of a wonderful small group at our church. The care we received was inspiring. We knew we were never alone."

Members of a small group can provide spiritual support with a personal touch. Here's what one person told me: "The members of my Sunday school class sent me cards, prayed for me during visits and phone calls, and sat with me during chemo when family members couldn't."

A key element of spiritual community is a sense of belonging, which small groups can provide. A woman said, "At the time of my cancer, I was in a circle of young women about my age. When I couldn't drive, they picked me up and took me to church. When I felt isolated, they provided hugs, comfort, and the assurance that I was still accepted and valued as part of the group."

Prayer within a small group can give real comfort. One survivor noted:

"Praying on my own was sometimes difficult and frustrating—at times I felt like the only answer I got was silence. But when I was with my group, all the shared prayers gave me a sense of peace and well-being. Praying with them lightened my load and made me feel like part of something bigger. It was God at work."

Large-Group Spiritual Community

It can also help to be part of a larger spiritual community—perhaps a congregation or other gathering. This kind of community can be a great place to find care, kindred spirits, and prayer support.

Care

People with cancer, as well as their loved ones, have shared with me many examples of the care they received from larger spiritual communities.

The spouse of a survivor said, "We had a steady flow of visits, prayers, and food from our church family. Everyone was incredibly supportive. We felt God's love through them—they were God's hands, voice, and face to us."

A woman said:

"A few months after we had moved across the country, our eight-year-old son was diagnosed with leukemia. Although we were new members of a congregation, they embraced us as though we'd been there for years. Parents of small children regularly volunteered to care for our four-year-old daughter, while other folks provided transportation or meals and helped with household chores or yard work. I don't know how we would've made it through that time without them."

Kindred Spirits

Another benefit of a large-group spiritual community is that you may find others who have had similar experiences. One man told me, "Some of the best supporters I found were other men from my church who'd had cancer." You can connect with these kindred spirits and benefit from their experience, understanding, and support (see chapter 64, "Find Kindred Spirits").

Prayer Support

Large-group spiritual communities are also a great source of prayer power. A number of people have told me how meaningful it was to have members of their spiritual community praying for them.

One person recalled:

> "During the first days after my diagnosis, I couldn't pray. Praying seemed to make it all too real, and I would get upset and panicky. But I was comforted by knowing that others from my church were already praying for me."

Another said:

> "The canopy of prayer that my congregation spread over me was the most important support I received. Knowing that the people on the congregation's prayer chain were praying for me every day gave me a peace that I wouldn't otherwise have had."

A woman shared:

> "My congregation gave me a prayer shawl. The woman who made it told me she had prayed for me the whole time she was knitting it. I'd put on that shawl during low times, and I'd wear it to stay warm during chemo. It helped me remember that I was being blanketed by the prayers of others. It gave me comfort and hope."

This point has come up a number of times in the book, but it can't be overstated: *You don't have to go it alone.* That's just as true when it comes to spiritual matters. A survivor summarized it well by saying, "I would greatly encourage anyone facing cancer to seek out spiritual community. It can make all the difference in the world—it certainly did for me."

Part 12

Giving Back

73

Pay It Forward

*"Having gone through the experience of cancer,
I have an idea of what to expect and what kinds
of help people may need. I've been there, and
now I can be of help to others."*

People may support you and your family in a variety of ways as you deal with cancer. You may sometimes wonder how you can ever repay them for all they've done. One good way is to pay it forward—to help others affected by cancer.

A survivor told me how it felt to pass along the care and support he had received:

"My friends and people at my job helped me out so much. I really felt their support in a powerful way, and it made me want to help others. So from time to time, I've talked with folks who were recently diagnosed, mainly just listening to them. They've said it helps them, and I've found that reaching out to others lifts my spirit too."

You don't have to pay it forward right away. The thought of doing so may seem daunting at first, especially when you are still dealing with cancer yourself. You might need to focus on your own situation for now. But when you feel ready, you may want to look for opportunities to help others.

Ways to Pay It Forward

Here are some possibilities for paying it forward.

Share your experience. At times, you may be able to share insights from your experience. Everyone's situation will be different, of course, but if someone asks for your thoughts or if something seems likely to apply to the other person, go ahead and share.

A woman told me:

> "A member of our church had the same kind of cancer I'd had and asked if we could talk. I met her for lunch, and after listening to her concerns and fears, I told her that I'd been in much the same place, and her thoughts and feelings were normal. Then I briefly mentioned a couple of insights I'd gained. She told me later that she appreciated our conversation and that it really helped her out."

Be a kindred spirit. Others may appreciate your offering comfort and support as a kindred spirit. A woman who'd had breast cancer said, "When other women tell me they have breast cancer, I give them a hug, say that I've been there, listen to them, and answer their questions about what it's like. I don't spend a lot of time sharing my own story; instead, I let them tell *their* story and get their feelings out." A man whose young son had cancer said, "At times, I'll learn about another dad whose son or daughter has been diagnosed. When that happens, I go out of my way to let him know I'm available to talk and support him however I can."

Offer the kinds of help that you really appreciated when you were dealing with cancer. You'll have a good idea of the kinds of help that were most valuable for you—or that you wish you'd had more of. Offering similar kinds of help to others can be a great way to pay it forward. One woman said, "I know what it's like to lose all your hair during treatment, so I'm always glad to help others pick out a nice wig or hat. Their smiles are priceless—helping to bring them a bit of joy in this difficult time is a beautiful thing."

Offer other kinds of practical help. You may have benefited from practical, nuts-and-bolts help in areas such as rides, childcare, housework, errand-running, or mowing your lawn. You may want to find ways to offer such practical help to others. If you aren't sure what kind of help someone needs, you can always ask.

Join with others to help those with cancer. Volunteering with a group that assists others with cancer can be a meaningful way to make a difference. One survivor told me, "I joined a group that makes soft, comfortable caps for people who lose their hair." Another said, "I volunteer with Reach to Recovery through the American Cancer Society." Still another noted, "I'm part of a team that drives people to their treatments."

Volunteer to speak with individuals or groups. A survivor talked about his experience: "A few times friends have said, 'Will you call so-and-so? He's getting ready to have surgery, and it would really help him to talk to someone who's been through it.' I've done this, and it feels good to be able to help someone else." Another said, "A year or so after I finished treatment and my cancer was in remission, a nurse asked me to speak to a support group. I decided to give it a try, and I'm glad I did. The people there really appreciated hearing my story. It gave them hope to go on."

There are many other ways you can help people dealing with cancer. Find something that fits your gifts and abilities and brings you joy and satisfaction. If you think of a way to help that makes you light up inside, it's probably right for you.

A Serendipity

One of life's serendipities, which I've witnessed countless times, is this: *When people give of themselves, they also receive.* When you reach out to others who are affected by cancer, they aren't the only ones who will benefit—you will, too.

74

Become
an Advocate

*"I've been a regular participant in our local cancer
fundraising event for several years. It's exciting and
empowering to be around so many other survivors.
We're helping to find a cure or develop better prevention
so others won't have to go through what we did."*

S omewhere down the line, you might find yourself thinking something
like, *I've been focused on my own fight for a while. Now I'd like to do something more to help prevent this disease and make things a little easier for others.
Maybe I can even play a small role in defeating cancer once and for all.*

If you ever have thoughts like these, you might want to consider becoming
an advocate.

Some cancer survivors, as well as loved ones, make advocacy a part of
their lives. The feeling of being a part of something bigger than yourself
can be extremely gratifying, especially when it's helping to defeat cancer.
It can provide a sense of community, accomplishment, and hope. One
person said, "Getting involved with the National Coalition for Cancer
Survivorship helped me see that I can do something about cancer on a
larger scale. It gives me hope that my children and grandchildren can live
free from this disease."

It may be a while before you feel ready to get involved in advocacy. Most
people wait until their treatments are over and they're feeling better before
they even start to think about it.

How Advocacy Is Different from Paying It Forward

Advocacy as defined in this chapter is different from what I described in the previous chapter, "Pay It Forward."

Paying it forward is helping individuals or small groups by offering them personal support and sharing firsthand experience. The emphasis is more direct—helping specific people who are affected by cancer.

Advocacy, on the other hand, involves helping in the broader fight against cancer, often working with larger organizations in more public efforts to bring about widespread change. It's about becoming part of a local, national, or global movement.

Both can be very effective and meaningful ways to give something back, but each does so on a different level.

Types of Advocacy Activities

You can find many ways to be an advocate, individually or with an organization. The American Cancer Society is probably the best-known cancer organization, but there are many others, often focused on a particular kind of cancer. You may even want to work with an organization that helped you.

Here are three ways that people commonly get involved as advocates.

1. Raising Money

Many organizations host events where cancer advocates can participate and help raise funds to support the cause.

- One person shared, "After I'd fully recovered from my surgery, I began participating in the American Cancer Society's Relay for Life. I've found it personally meaningful because I want to help find a cure or prevent cancer however I can. Fundraising is a tangible way I can support the cause."

- Another survivor volunteered at a local cancer association to help coordinate fundraising efforts. "I help raise money that goes to the patients with the greatest needs in our community," she said. "What a blessing it is to help provide essential support for so many people!"

- A breast cancer survivor joined with her friends to participate in a fundraising walk for cancer treatment, and afterward they were determined to do more. She told me, "We set up an annual event that raises money to provide mammograms for women who can't afford them. Almost 20 years later, it's still going strong!"

- One man shared that he and a group of other testicular cancer survivors participated in races and other local fundraising events to support research and build awareness.

- A mother whose son survived cancer said, "Every year my son and I host an 'Ice Cream for Breakfast' fundraiser and donate the proceeds to children's cancer organizations. It's an important way both of us can say thank you for the support and care we received. My son's still young, but he's already become quite an advocate."

Whether you participate in an existing fundraising event or organize one yourself, there are many chances to help raise money for the cause.

2. Political Involvement

Getting involved politically may mean joining a cancer advocacy group that's active in lobbying or letter writing. You can also conduct your own campaign of calling, writing, or emailing elected officials to tell them your views and encourage them to support cancer-related policies and legislation.

- One person said, "I've signed up to receive notifications whenever a bill related to cancer research or treatment is coming up in Congress. When one comes up that I believe in, I do everything I can to get the word out and urge my representatives to support it."

- Several people told me they've traveled to their state capital or to Washington, D.C., to participate in rallies to build awareness and support increased funding for cancer research.

- Others have volunteered with the American Cancer Society Cancer Action Network (ACS CAN). They received training and tools to advocate for local, state, or national legislation that affects the well-being of cancer patients and their families. Some send letters or email, talk with legislators, or speak before legislative committees. One said, "Through ACS CAN, I've worked with many dedicated people in helping to pass meaningful legislation on the state and national level. I've had the chance to meet cancer patients, concerned citizens, and legislators. It's opened up a whole new world to me."

Political progress may take a while, but if enough people speak up, it can happen, potentially making a huge difference against cancer overall.

3. Raising Awareness

A third means of advocacy is to help others learn about cancer. Because cancer is such a misunderstood, frightening topic for many people, a little understanding can go a long way to help clear up misconceptions, encourage preventive practices, or generally boost awareness.

Writing, speaking, distributing pamphlets, staffing a booth—you can get the word out in many ways.

- One person said she volunteers at her hospital's cancer resource center, handing out information on programs and support groups.

- A melanoma survivor told me that he speaks frequently at various groups in the community, encouraging people to practice sun safety.

- A breast cancer survivor wrote an article for the local newspaper, telling her story and encouraging others to get mammograms. Afterward, she heard from a number of women who'd acted on her advice. "That's just the response I was hoping for," she told me. "Some of them jokingly told me it was 'all my fault' that they got a mammogram. I'll gladly take the blame, since it means lives will be saved."

- A colon cancer survivor conducting his own awareness campaign said, "I'm a crusader for early detection. I encouraged one friend to get a colonoscopy, and he found cancer early. His medical team successfully treated it, and now he's gotten back to the business of living to a ripe old age. Knowing I can make a difference like that makes it all worthwhile."

Being involved in awareness-building efforts is a way to personally help people detect cancer early—or perhaps avoid it entirely.

Whether or not you become involved in advocacy is up to you. But if you think you might be interested and the timing feels right, consider what area of advocacy may best fit your abilities and comfort level. By becoming an advocate, you can experience the satisfaction of knowing that you're helping make life better for countless others—those who will face cancer after you, and those who may never have to, due in part to your efforts.

Chronological Diagnosis and Treatment Tracking Tools

This appendix describes and includes samples of two tools you can adapt for tracking your medical history.

1. **Chronological Diagnosis and Treatment Summary.** This summary provides a historical record of medical activity from the initial diagnosis to the present. You can assemble this information from various sources, including what your oncologist tells you, test results, imaging reports, pathology reports, surgical reports, and other sources.

2. **Chronological Diagnosis and Treatment Calendar.** This calendar provides a snapshot of your treatment to date, pulling highlights from the summary and giving a clear overview at a glance.

Both the summary and the calendar can be valuable for tracking and communicating the overall course of your treatment. You and your loved ones can use them to easily verify what happened at a particular point in your treatment. These two tools can be useful for updating a medical professional who might not be familiar with every aspect of your treatment; he or she can look at the calendar to quickly trace your history with cancer and then refer back to the summary for more details.

You Don't Need to Do It All

You can choose how much information to track and whether to ask for help tracking it.

Throughout your treatment, you may gather a lot of information to possibly include in your summary and calendar. You don't need to keep track of everything—just focus on what you think would be most helpful and what you're comfortable doing.

Also, if you don't feel up to doing this yourself, you might ask a friend or family member with organizational skills to help you. A man whose wife had cancer talked about using these tools: "I can't really help my wife medically since I'm not a doctor—but this is something I *can* do. And I know it's helpful because a couple of times at an appointment, one of her doctors has asked about something, and I've been able to quickly find the information that was needed."

Information You Might Include

Here are suggestions for what kinds of information you might include in your summary and calendar. Much of this information can be taken directly from the reports and other information you receive from your medical team.

Diagnosis. This is the full diagnosis your oncologist gave you, including the specific type and stage of the cancer.

Surgery. This includes the type of surgery, the name of the surgeon, the date of the surgery, and the facility where the surgery took place. If you have a copy of the operative report for your surgery or the pathology report, you might mention that.

Treatment Plan. It's helpful to describe the overall plan of treatment (such as radiation or chemotherapy), including the number of treatments, the names and dosages of medication(s) to be used, and the facility where the treatments will take place.

Individual Treatments. You can have a separate entry for each time you receive a treatment, identifying the type of treatment and possibly including the names and dosages of medication(s) used, the date of the treatment, the facility where the treatment took place, and anything notable that occurred during or following the treatment.

Lab Work. You can record any information on lab work used to help track the effectiveness of your treatment, including what was tracked (for instance, a tumor marker), its level on each date, and the facility where the level was checked.

Imaging. This includes the type of image taken (such as X-ray or CT scan), the area of the body, what the image showed, the date the image was taken, and the facility where it was taken. If you have a copy of a report or an image—whether hard copy or digital copy—you might note that.

Test or Procedure. When you have a test or procedure performed, you can record its name, the area of the body, the result, the date it occurred, the facility where the test or procedure took place, and the name of the physician.

Office Visit. For each office visit, it's helpful to list the name of the physician, the physician's specialty, the date of the visit, and any significant topics discussed—such as managing pain, dealing with side effects, or exploring treatment options. Note any changes to your medications.

As you can see, there's a lot of information you could incorporate into your summary and calendar—but again, you don't need to do it all. Adapt these ideas to fit your needs; you might decide to keep track of fewer kinds of information, include different details, or format the information in a different way.

The goal is to keep track of your personal medical information in a way that works well for you. Having an easy-to-access summary of your medical history can improve communication with medical professionals, enhance your sense of control over your treatment, and help you feel more confident.

The following pages show a fictional example of each tool, describing a few months' worth of treatment, to give you an idea of how all this information might fit together. Note that your own summary or calendar would most likely include a higher level of detail than these examples do. Also, since each person's situation is unique, the specifics in these examples may be very different from your own course of treatment.

1. Chronological Diagnosis and Treatment Summary

FICTIONAL EXAMPLE

The purpose of this example is to give you an idea of the types of events and details to include in your own summary. Since every person and situation is different, the specifics in this example may not reflect every patient's experience, including those with colon cancer.

[Patient's Name]

5/13/XX

Office visit with Dr. A (internist) to describe symptoms (diarrhea and discolored stool). Test of stool sample revealed blood in the stool. Referred to Dr. B (gastroenterologist) for colonoscopy.

5/27/XX

Memorial Hospital. Dr. B (gastroenterologist). Colonoscopy. Lesion identified and biopsied. Tissue sent to pathologist.

6/5/XX

Memorial Hospital. Dr. B (gastroenterologist). See pathology report. Cancer is [type of cancer]. CT scan scheduled. Referred to Dr. C (surgeon).

6/9/XX

Memorial Hospital. CT scan.

6/12/XX

Memorial Hospital. Dr. C (surgeon). Discussed CT scan results. See report and film. Surgery scheduled.

6/17/XX

Memorial Hospital. Dr. C (surgeon). Surgery [include details of surgery]. See operative report. Tissue sent to pathologist.

6/24/XX

Memorial Hospital. Dr. C (surgeon). The cancer is [type and stage of cancer]. Two lymph nodes were cancerous. See pathology report. Referred to Dr. D (medical oncologist) to determine treatment.

7/22/XX

Oncology Center. Office visit with Dr. D (medical oncologist) to discuss treatment options. Treatment plan determined.

Plan of treatment

[Description of treatment plan]

7/29/XX

Oncology Center. Treatment #1.

8/12/XX

Oncology Center. Treatment #2.

8/26/XX

Oncology Center. Treatment #3.

2. Chronological Diagnosis and Treatment Calendar

FICTIONAL EXAMPLE

The purpose of this example is to give you an idea of the types of events and details to include in your own calendar. Since every person and situation is different, the specifics in this example may not reflect every patient's experience, including those with colon cancer.

[Patient's Name]

May 20XX

Date	Treatment	Lab Work	Imaging	Office Visit	Surgery, Test, or Procedure
5/13				Dr. A (internist).	Dr. A's office. Test for blood in stool. Test showed blood in stool.
5/27					Memorial Hospital. Dr. B (gastroenterologist). Colonoscopy. Lesion identified and biopsied. See report.

June 20XX

Date	Treatment	Lab Work	Imaging	Office Visit	Surgery, Test, or Procedure
6/5				Memorial Hospital. Dr. B (gastroen-terologist).	

Date	Treatment	Lab Work	Imaging	Office Visit	Surgery, Test, or Procedure
6/5				*continued* Pathology report. Cancer is [type of cancer]. CT scan scheduled.	
6/9			Memorial Hospital. CT scan.		
6/12				Memorial Hospital. Dr. C (surgeon). See report and film. Surgery scheduled.	
6/17					Memorial Hospital. Dr. C (surgeon). Surgery [include details of surgery]. See operative report.
6/24				Memorial Hospital. Dr. C (surgeon). Pathology report. Cancer is [type and stage of cancer.]	

July 20XX

Date	Treatment	Lab Work	Imaging	Office Visit	Surgery, Test, or Procedure
7/22				Oncology Center. Dr. D (medical oncologist). Treatment plan determined.	
7/29	Oncology Center. Treatment #1.				

August 20XX

Date	Treatment	Lab Work	Imaging	Office Visit	Surgery, Test, or Procedure
8/12	Oncology Center. Treatment #2.				
8/26	Oncology Center. Treatment #3.				

THANK YOU

Thank you for allowing me to walk with you during this time. I would be deeply gratified if you've found help, hope, and comfort in this book.

Because everyone's story is unique, I always appreciate hearing from readers like you. If this book has helped you in some way and you'd like to share your thoughts, insights, or experiences, please write to me about them. I would welcome your comments.

God bless you.

ABOUT THE AUTHOR

Kenneth C. Haugk is a psychologist, author, pastor, and teacher. He received his Ph.D. in clinical psychology from Washington University and his M.Div. from Concordia Seminary, both in St. Louis, Missouri. A member of the American Psychological Association, he has served as a clinical psychologist and has taught psychology and counseling at several universities and seminaries.

Dr. Haugk is the founder and Executive Director of Stephen Ministries in St. Louis. He is the author of a number of books, including *Speaking the Truth in Love, When and How to Use Mental Health Resources,* and *Don't Sing Songs to a Heavy Heart: How to Relate to Those Who Are Suffering,* and has published widely in psychological journals and popular periodicals. He is a frequent conference and workshop speaker.

When Ken's wife, Joan—a registered nurse, social worker, and mother—was diagnosed with ovarian cancer, they began a three-and-a-half-year battle against the disease. Together, they navigated the medical, emotional, relational, and spiritual challenges that can come when dealing with cancer.

Bringing together his personal and professional experience, Ken wrote *Cancer—Now What?* as a resource people can give to help others address the challenges of cancer. He conducted research with thousands of cancer survivors, their loved ones, and medical professionals, incorporating their wisdom and expertise in the book.

Ken lives in St. Louis, where he enjoys playing basketball, watching baseball, and spending time with his two daughters, son-in-law, and two grandchildren.